NEW MEDICAL FRONTIERS, INC.

>>><<<

BOOK
OF
NATURAL HEALTH
Your Source of Health & Longevity

Volume 4

50 chapters, scientifically validated

Dr. Mark Fritz, NMD, PhD

>>><<<

Copyright © Dr. Mark Fritz, New Medical Frontiers, Inc. 2023

ISBN: 9798375574011

All rights reserved.
No part of this publication may be reproduced, stored in a retrieval system, or transmitted, in any form or by any means, electronic, mechanical, photocopying, recording, or otherwise, without the written prior permission of the author.

DISCLAIMER

The content of this book is for informational purposes only and is not intended to replace the advice and treatment by a healthcare provider. Every metabolism is different. Work with your physician/healthcare provider to find the best solutions for your heath.

All contents of this book are commentary or opinion and are protected under Free Speech Laws in all civilized countries. The information is provided for educational and entertainment purposes only and is not intended to diagnose, treat, cure, or prevent any condition or disease. Dr. Mark Fritz assumes no responsibility for the use or misuse of this material. No warranty of any kind, whether expressed or implied, is given in relation to this information or any of the external services referred to. This is a comprehensive limitation of liability that applies to all damages of any kind, including (without limitation) compensatory, direct, indirect or consequential damages.

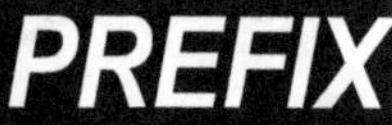

PREFIX

This is the 4th volume of the series "Books of Natural Health" for citizens and patients, who understand that they themselves are primarily responsible for their most precious good in life – their health – which, to be sure, is based on laws of nature.

Doing justice accordingly, 2 avenues to make use of this book best:

- Read it from chapter 1-50 for your information/education.
- Look up more 300 health issues, remedies and modalities listed in alphabetical order in 'Index' to find natural answers to a specific health problem.

See exact scientific validations by more than 400 U.S. and international universities/medical schools and research institutions – all listed in alphabetical order at the end in 'references'.

Dr. Mark Fritz, NMD, PhD
President
of
New Medical Frontiers, Inc.

A leading independent documentation & information center for latest scientific breakthroughs in natural/naturopathic medicine on a global basis

www.newmedicalfrontiers.com

CONTENTS

Instead of an own

FOREWORD

"If people let government decide what food they eat and what medicine they take, their bodies will soon be in as sorry a state as are the souls of those who live under tyranny."

American President Thomas Jefferson
("Man of the People")
1743-1826

1. OVERWEIGHT? MIND YOUR MEDICATIONS!

THE PHILOSOPHY BEHIND

According to the U.S. governmental Centers for Disease Control and Prevention (CDC) two thirds of our adult population are overweight, half of those even obese. With manifold consequences of debilitating diseases, heart failure and cancer included, and even premature death.

Besides genetics which applies to roughly one percent of cases, causes behind of this seemingly vicious cycle are basically unhealthy diet and lack of physical exercise. Period? Not really. There is in fact one more major cause behind most citizens have never heard and – unfortunately – have not been informed about by their healthcare provider: certain synthetic medications can cause weight gain as one of its manifold side effects. Not necessarily with first drug administration but even after some months or years of regular drug swallowing.

By, inter alia, altering the metabolism of our body as well as influencing electrolyte and water balances. Or due to changes in mood, increasing appetite which may even cause cravings. Also, shortness of breath due to certain medications makes it harder to exercise.

SCIENTIFIC VERIFICATION

This may especially happen with respect to following medications, regardless if on prescription or OTC:

- Opioids
- Antipsychotics and mood stabilizers
- Antidepressants
- Epilepsy medications
- Diabetes medications
- Corticosteroids
- Beta-blockers

Based on research at, inter alia, the
- *Obesity Medicine Association* in Denver, CO,
- *Arizona State University* in Mesa, AZ
- *American Academy of Child and Adolescent Psychiatry* in Washington, D.C.
- *King's College London & Guy's Hospital* (both London, UK)

as well as the Canadian scientific institutions
- *University of Ottawa* and *Children's Hospital of Eastern Ontario* in Ottawa
- *Mcgill University* in Montreal
- *University of Toronto* in Toronto
- *University of Calgary* in Calgary
- *Laval University* in Quebec City and
- *Western University* in London, Ontario

NATURE'S ANSWER

While this may sound as a vicious cycle, since most citizens take some kind of synthetic medication more or less regularly – no it is not. Because of the fact that not only our planet the Earth, but also our body is a biologic-ecologic phenomenon strictly based on natural laws – yes, nature gives us remedies without any negative side effects for our health. Scientifically validated by contemporary medical science.

Therefore, in case of any health issue, just ask us about appropriate natural remedies to replace synthetic drugs.

IN A NUTSHELL

In most cases, reasons of being overweight or even obese are unhealthy diet and a sedentary lifestyle. Manifold leading to debilitating health issues. Now we learn from medical science that also many ordinary synthetic medications may cause weight problems. Fortunately, you can break this vicious cycle with natural alternatives. Scientifically verified.

2. SUFFER MAJOR DEPRESSION DISORDER?

THE PHILOSOPHY BEHIND

Depression is one of the debilitating health issues of our 'modern' times, effecting one out of six citizens once in a lifetime. Potentially caused by psychological, biological or environmental reasons. One severe and maybe least understood kind is 'clinical' depression as a major depressive mood disorder.

TYPES OF CLINICAL DEPRESSION – SCIENTIFICALLY VERIFIED

Based on research at, inter alia

- *University of Cincinnati* in Cincinnati, OH
- *University of Pittsburgh* in Pittsburgh, PA
- *Iowa State University* in Ames, IA
- *Sichuan University/West China Hospital* in Chengdu, China
- *Chonnam National University Medical School* in Gwangju, South Korea
- *Hwasun Hospital* in Hwasun, South Korea
- *University of Genoa* in Genoa, Italy
- *Universita degli Studi della Campagnia 'Luigi Vanvitelli'* in Napoli, Italy
- *Universidad Nacional de Educacion a Distancia (UNED)* in Spain
- *Universita degli Studi di Cagliari* in Cagliari, Italy

there are basically 3 different types of clinical depression:

- Major depression with seasonal pattern
  (E.g., in winter time, lacking sunshine)
- Major depression disorder with peripartum onset
  (Up to 6% of women may experience this episode during pregnancy or first year after delivery)
- Major depressive disorder with psychotic features
  (Inter alia, experiencing delusions or hallucinations)

Along with symptoms, depending on age, as follows:

- *Age 6-17*
  Potential symptoms (inter alia):

- Physical aches and pain
- Difficulty to pay attention
- Feeling sad or depressed for several hours
- Feeling nervous/scared/anxious
- Having a vision while awake
- Hearing voices when no one is there
- Frequently feeling an urge to check on things
- Starting more projects or taking more risks
- Frequently concerned about health or feeling unwell
- Feeling a need to do something in a specific way to prevent anything bad from happening
- Having less fun than normal
- Having lots of energy with unusually little sleep
- Avoiding doing things because they cause nervousness
- Thinking of self or others doing something bad or having something bad happen
- Becoming easily annoyed or irritated
- Sleeping problems

Additionally, it may be checked if the respective young person has been involved in risky behaviors such as

- Smoking/snuffing/chewing tobacco
- Drugs (like cannabis, cocaine, ecstasy)
- Pharmaceutical medicine without prescription
- Thoughts of suicide
- Alcohol consumption

- *Adults (18+)*
  In this age bracket, symptoms usually include

- Feeling frightened/panicked
- Considering self-harm
- Avoiding situations causing anxiety
- Having sleep problems
- Experience separation from self/memory/ body/surroundings
- Feeling distance from others
- Smoking/snuffing/chewing tobacco
- Feeling others may hear own thoughts or vice versa
- Much energy despite less sleep
- Feeling irritated/angry/grouchy
- Experience physical pain with seemingly no cause
- Hearing things which others may not hear

- Consuming more alcohol than usual
- Feeling confused about self
- Kick off projects and risks more than usual
- Feeling low/hopeless
- Experience lack of interest/pleasure in certain activities
- Experience difficulty with orientation/memory
- Feeling anxious/nervous/scared
- Feeling a drive to complete mental/physical acts repeatedly
- Have recurring images/urges/unpleasant thoughts
- Feeling that others don't take own illness serious

NATURE'S ANSWER

Based on above mentioned research a healthy active lifestyle with special reference to vigorous

- *Physical exercise*

 may be nature's excellent recommendation to treat symptoms of depression and avoid related mortality best.

IN A NUTSHELL

Major depressive disorder (known also by the medical term *clinical depression*) is a severe mood disorder of different features, leading in some cases even to suicide. This however, can be counterbalanced by healthful active lifestyle. With special reference to physical activity.

3. COFFEE: GOOD OR BAD FOR HYPERTENSION?

THE PHILOSOPHY BEHIND

Coffee is one of the most conflicting foods for our health.

On one side, caffeine is a so called vasoconstrictor, i.e. it cuts down the size of blood vessels and accordingly, may increase blood pressure. By interacting with certain receptors in the brain. Vice versa, caffeine comprises antioxidants which can protect the blood vessels.

WHAT SCIENCE TELLS US ABOUT

Based on this seemingly conflicting situation, research at
- *University of Catania* in Catania, Italy
- *University of Navarra* and *Navarra's Health Research Institute* in Pamplona, Spain
  and
- *Jagiellonian University Medical College* in Krakow, Poland

concludes that drinking 7 cups of coffee per day decreases hypertension by 9%, adding 1% more decrease with any additional cup.

Along with additional protective effect of phenols in caffeine.

At least 3-4 cups of coffee per day may not be a problem for people with high blood pressure also according to research at the *University of Oklahoma College of Medicine* in Oklahoma City, OK.

On the other hand, with respect to research at the *Agricultural University of Athens* and *Attikon University Hospital,* both in Athens, Greece, as well as the *United Arab Emirates University* in El Ain, United Arab Emirates, caffeine does increase blood pressure – however, still within healthy ranges.

This may be seen in line with research at *Ohio State University* in Columbus, OH, and *Charite University Medical Center* in Berlin, Germany, according to which infrequent coffee may not be dangerous.

Only regular consumption of 1-3 cups regular per day may slightly increase hypertension, according to research at *Michigan State University* in East Lansing, MI.

IN A NUTSHELL

The scientific findings indicated above may seem conflicting and inconsistent at first glance, as far as coffee consumption is concerned with respect to blood pressure.

Still, summing up according to the *American College of Cardiology*, a consumption of up to 300 milligrams of caffeine per day may not only be safe with respect to blood pressure. It may also protect against heart rhythm disorders.

If you are still doubtful about coffee consumption, depending on your body's individual tolerance, you have at least the chance to replace caffeine with other gifts of nature such as, inter alia,
- *rooibos tea*
- *roasted barley or grain drinks*
- *yerba mate*
- *dandelion root coffee*
- *chicory coffee*

Especially in cases where coffee consumption may be related personally to, e.g., anxiety, insomnia, tremors or heartburn.

---

4. BRACE YOUR IMMUNITY NATURALLY

THE PHILOSOPHY BEHIND

To live a healthy and long life depends primarily on our inherent strong and powerful immune system. To ward off infections leading to chronic illness and premature death. While this is basic part of our existence, we still need to support our immune system during our whole life. Because the immune system not only is weakening over time, it also becomes imbalanced later in life.

This is true for both sides of our immune system – the *innate* immunity and the *adaptive* immunity.

The

Innate immunity

is important to avoid infections potentially leading otherwise to chronic inflammation such as, inter alia, cardiovascular disease, cancer, diabetes or dementia, and in autoimmune conditions like rheumatoid arthritis, etc.

On the other side, the

Adaptive immunity

recognizes/remembers and attacks/neutralizes particular pathogens to defend against bacteria, viruses, and fungi.

This part of our immune system has special reference later in life. Not only to avoid chronic illness and premature death by itself, a weak adaptive immunity also makes vaccinations less effective. This is also true for flu vaccinations which, if done repeatedly, could even lead to reduction of antibody responses.

NATURAL WAYS TO BOLSTER IMMUNITY – SCIENTIFICALLY VALIDATED

To strengthen the immune system the natural way also later in life, comprehensive international research recommends following lifestyle adjustments.

Physical exercise

On a regular basis, physical exercise is inevitable, according to research at, the
- *University of Houston* in Houston, TX
- *University of Birmingham* in Birmingham, UK
- *Edinburgh Napier University* in Edinburgh, UK
  and in Sao Paulo, Brazil, at the
- *University of Sao Paulo*
  and the
- *Clinics Hospital*

Because keeping skeleton muscles intact produces proteins named myokines which cut down inflammation and supports immunity. With special reference to health conditions such as cardiovascular disease and diabetes 2, which are strongly linked to chronic inflammation.

Mediterranean diet

Chances to avoid frailty with special reference to loss of muscle strength, walking slowly and getting easily tired are also linked to Mediterranean diet with special reference to, inter alia,
- large amounts of olive oil, leafy vegetable and fruit
- moderate amounts of fish, dairy and poultry
  and
- low amounts of added sugar and red meat
lowering also the risk of cardiovascular disease, cancer and diabetes 2.

Based on research at, inter alia, the
- *University College London* in London, UK
- *Catholic University Leuven* in Leuven, Belgium
- *Charles University* in Prague, Czechia
- *University of Sao Paulo* in Sao Paulo, Brazil
- *University of Bologna* in Bologna, Italy
  and the
- *Universidad Nacional Autonoma de Mexico* in Mexico City, Mexico

Weight management

is at the same time equally important, since up to 30% of the pro-inflammatory cytokine IL-6 to be found in the bloodstream come from adipose tissue, as a massive contributor to being overweight and obese, leading to chronic inflammation considerably.

According to research at, inter alia,
- *University of Miami School of Medicine* in Miami, FL
- *University of Innsbruck* in Innsbruck, Austria
- *University of Sherbrooke* in Sherbrooke, Canada
- *University of Modena and Reggio Emilia* in Modena, Italy
- *University Pierre & Marie Curie (Sorbonne University)* in Paris, France
- *University of Houston* in Houston, TX

IN A NUTSHELL

The most important natural tool for long and healthy life is our inherent immune system. Yet, it is important to support it by appropriate lifestyle factors regularly, to ward off chronic disease and premature death. Especially, the older we get. With special reference to both sides of the immune system – innate and adaptive immunity, as you have learned in this chapter.

5. ALICE IN WONDERLAND SYNDROME?

THE PHILOSOPHY BEHIND

In 1955, the English psychiatrist John Todd coined the term *Alice in Wonderland Syndrome (AIWS)* – also named "Todd's Syndrome" today. Based on the famous book "Alice's Adventures in Wonderland" by Lewis Carroll.

What stands behind of AIWS from a medical point of view?

In fact, it is the neurological key term for a situation where somebody may experience perceptual disorders which can affect this person's brain activity in terms of
- hearing
- sensation
- time
- touch
 or
- sight

TYPES OF AIWS - SCIENTIFICALLY VERIFIED

Although this syndrome is usually related to young people, it still occurs in all age groups.

Thereby, we differ between 3 main types of AIWS depending on the respective perceptual disorder:

- A - Disorders being somesthetic/sensory
- B - Affecting visual senses
- C - Mix of A & B

Based on international research at, inter alia,
- *State University of New York* in Buffalo, NY
- *Tomah VA Medical Center* in Tomah, WI
- *Centre Hospitaliser Universitaire Vaudois* in Lausanne, Switzerland
- *University of Groningen* in Groningen, The Netherlands

While category "A" includes people who feel as though their body parts are changing size, category "B" is causing more visual distortions of the surrounding environment, such as

- *micropsia*, where the respective person is seeing objects smaller than their actual size;
- *macropsia* with objects being seemingly too big;
- *teleopsia* for objects being seemingly farther away than they really are;
- *pelopsia* with objects
  or
- *metamorphopsia* when shapes of objects like width or height seem to be inaccurate

Category "C" applies for people feeling that their own body and/or other persons or stuff around them is changing.

Related to certain symptoms including, inter alia
- distorted body image or perception of size
- altered perception of time
- metamorphopsia
- feverish symptoms
- epileptic seizures affecting part of the brain
- migraine episodes

Thereby, AIWS may be caused by certain diseases such as, inter alia,
- lyme neuroborreliosis
- scarlet fever/tonsillopharyngitis (streptococcus pyogenes)
- mycoplasma
- influenza A virus
- typhoid encephalopathy
- varicella-zoster virus
  as well as
- medication
- psychiatric conditions
- epilepsy
- stroke
- brain lesions
- head trauma

With migraines and Epstein-Barr virus infections being the most common AIWS causes.

However, also brain tumors may cause AIWS at least temporarily, according to research at the *Medical and Finance Center* in Gronau, Germany

IN A NUTSHELL

Patterned on Lewis Carrol's book "Alice's Adventures in Wonderland", *Alice in Wonderland Syndrome (AIWS)* is a disorienting neurological health issue. Causing perceptual disorders, as how the brain may perceive things, changing temporarily. Coined 1955 by the English psychiatrist John Todd (therefore, AIWS is also known by the term "Todd's Syndrome").

6. FIGHT CANCER WITH HONEYBEES?

THE PHILOSOPHY BEHIND

According to latest medical statistics of the World Health Organization (WHO), in the industrialized world 86% of non-age-related deaths are the consequence of seemingly 'chronic' – yet widely preventable – diseases. With heart failure on top of the chart. Followed by cancer as # 2. Half a century after former U.S. president Nixon had declared the 'War on Cancer' in 1971.

This implies that chemotherapy and radiation as the prime therapy of conventional oncology, only can put the cancer patient on remission – without a cure.

In fact, the only way to cure cancer successfully may be found in nature. Where and what in nature?

HONEYBEE VENOM AS THE SCIENTIFICALLY VERIFIED ANSWER?

Only recently, 2 renowned Chinese medical research institutions – the
- *Fourth Military Medical University* in the city of Xi'an
  and the
- *Beijing Institute for Brain Disorders* in China's capital Beijing

have found in laboratory studies that a major component of the honeybee venom killed breast cancer cells. Particularly triple-negative breast cancer cells.

With similar benefits also for lung, ovarian, pancreatic and melanoma cancers.

Destroying cancer cell membranes within 60 minutes – without harming healthy cells.

Scientifically validated in Australia at the *University of Western Australia* and the *Harry Perkins Institute of Medical Research,* both in Perth.

This venom is *melittin,* a molecule which also creates the painful sensation of a bee's sting.

Although seeming 'revolutionary', these findings may not be really surprising when we appreciate the fact that man has used honey, propolis and venom from the European honeybee *Apis mellifera* for health since thousands of years.

IN A NUTSHELL

According to research in laboratory tests at 2 renowned medical institutions in China, and scientifically verified by 2 medical institutions in Australia, a component of honeybee venom named *melittin* may be capable to kill cancer cells successfully. Easily available on the market, at a reasonable price. Unlike chemotherapy and radiation which costs a fortune, without a cure.

7. BENEFITS OF PEPPERMINT OIL FOR HEALTH

THE PHILOSOPHY BEHIND

As you have learned from our previous scientifically validated publications, to support good health and long life, nature gives us unlimited power. With special reference to herbs. One of most powerful plants is peppermint, a hybrid of spearmint and water mint, well known for centuries to treat health issues. Containing more than 40 compounds including *menthol*.

SCIENTIFICALLY VERIFIED BENEFITS OF PEPPERMINT OIL

Peppermint oil is derived from the peppermint plant as an essential oil. Available in different forms such as,
- highly concentrated pure
- less concentrated extract
and
- enteric-coated capsules

Usually used in aromatherapy to be applied to the skin or inhaled through steam of diffuser.

However, while healthcare providers are warning to take this oil orally in concentrated pure form, as it may be toxic in high doses, it is appreciated in traditional herbalism for different health benefits like, inter alia,
- pain relief
- boosting blood circulation
- killing germs/viruses
- etc,
scientifically validated today.

Inter alia,

- *Reducing Irritable Bowel Syndrome (IBS) symptoms*

such as abdominal pain, frequent bouts of diarrhea and constipation, as an enteric-coated diluted oil.

According to research at, inter alia,
- *Johns Hopkins University School of Medicine* in Baltimore, MD
- *King Saud University* in Riyad, Saudi Arabia

and
- *University of Mohaghegh Ardabili* in Ardabil, Iran
by blocking movement of calcium across intestinal membrane.

Another benefit may be

- *Easing nausea and vomiting*

by inhaling peppermint oil vapor especially when recovering from heart surgery. Based on research at *Kashan University of Medical Sciences* in Kashan, Iran.

- *Antiviral activity*

With special reference to *herpes simplex* viruses and *influenza type A* viruses. Based on research at, inter alia, the *University of Agriculture and Technology* in Orissa, India.

Also, peppermint oil may relief effectively from

- *Chronic Itching*

according to the *National Research Centre* in Egypt's capital Cairo.

Additionally, peppermint oil has been identified as an improvement for

- *Athletic performance*

like grip strength and jumping. Based on research at, inter alia, the *University of Mohaghegh Ardabili* in Ardabil, Iran.

LIMITS

Although the benefits of peppermint oil are scientifically verified, pure and highly concentrated essential peppermint oils may be toxic. With menthol potentially causing side effects especially in children.

IN A NUTSHELL

Peppermint oil is just one example of powerful herbal remedy we find in the unlimited kingdom of nature for our health which has been used for centuries by our ancestors with certain limits, and which has been scientifically validated today.

8. RELIEVE PSORIATIC ARTHRITIS NATURALLY

THE PHILOSOPHY BEHIND

Although not life-endangering, psoriatic arthritis (PsA) is definitely one of the most debilitating health issues of our modern times. With symptoms of pain, inflammation and swelling of the joints.

NATURE'S ANSWER SCIENTIFICALLY VALIDATED

While you can relieve these symptoms with pharmaceutical drugs – all along with side effects – there are quite a few remedies and modalities to cope with PsA softly the natural way.

Remedies

- *Omega-3*

Based on research at *Mt. San Jacinto College* in San Jacinto, CA, this constituent of fish oil (as we find it in oily cold-water fish such as tuna, etc.) may well ease inflammation and painful swelling, accordingly.

- *Turmeric*

More precise, what we are focusing on here is *curcumin,* the gold colored anti-inflammatory constituent of the herb turmeric which in fact has been documented already 2000 years ago in the Holy Bible.

To be self-medicated as a spice or with turmeric capsules.

Based on research, inter alia, at *Texas Southern University* in Houston, TX, and the *University of Miami* in Florida.

- *Ginger*

According to research of the U.S. *Arthritis Foundation* in Atlanta, GA, ginger is another beneficial herb (root) to help not only with PsA, but also *rheumatic* arthritis, because of its anti-inflammatory properties.

- *Capsaicin*

This constituent of chili peppers, available on the market as a cream, may relieve pain in the joints.
According to research at, inter alia, *Imperial College London* in the UK.

Modalities

- *Acupuncture*

You can insert needles at certain pressure points to relieve chronic pain.

Based on research at, inter alia, the *University of Miami* in Florida.

- *Exercise*

According to research at, inter alia, the *University of Alabama* in Birmingham, AL, low-impact physical activities like swimming may well help people with PsA.

- *Epsom salts*

A warm bath with epsom salts may well relieve inflammation and pain of the joints, as it contains the mineral *magnesium* for better bone health.

Besides of the fact that warm water with temperature between 92 and 100 degrees Fahrenheit (33 – 38 degrees Celsius) anyhow can loosen joints and also relieve joint pain.

Based on research at, inter alia, *Dewpoint Therapeutics* in Dresden, Germany.

- *Avoid/quit smoking*

since this un-natural habit can well trigger PsA and flares of symptoms.

According to research at, inter alia, the *University of Alabama* in Birmingham, AL.

IN A NUTSHELL

Psoriatic arthritis, a debilitating health issue with pain, inflammation and swelling of joints, is naturally treatable. With certain remedies and modalities our ancestors have used already centuries ago. As focused on in this chapter, scientifically validated.

9. RIGHT DIET FOR HEALTH & LONGEVITY

THE PHILOSOPHY BEHIND

Our health and longevity rests basically on 2 pillars: physical activity and healthy diet. Since millions of years, when man entered this globe.

Leaving us with the question which foods are – and which are not – only tasty but also the most appropriate ones to support health and longevity. Because of their nutrients.

While those appropriate foods are unlimited available on our planet in terms of quantity and quality, we shall focus at least on a small variety in following.

Vegetables

Based on research at, inter alia, *Tuskegee University* in Tuskegee, AL,

- *Spinach*

is highly valuable because of its vital nutrients such as

- Vitamins A/B-3/B-6/C/E/K
- Calcium
- Potassium
- Selenium
- Zinc
- Betaine
- Phosphor
- Copper
- Iron
- Manganese

Also

- *Broccoli*

is highly efficient because of its content of

- Potassium

- Folate
- Calcium
- Fiber
- Vitamin C
- Beta-carotene
  and
- Phytonutrients (reducing the risk of heart disease, diabetes, cancer)
  as well as
- Sulforaphane (fighting inflammation and cancer)

According to research at, inter alia, the *University of Heidelberg* in Heidelberg, Germany.

- *Kale*

as another green leafy vegetable is very potent because of its content of

- Vitamins C & K.

According to the *U.S. Department of Agriculture.*

- *Sweet potatoes*

According to the U.S. *Center for Science in the Public Interest* in Washington, D.C., sweet potatoes are very beneficial because of their

- Vitamins A & C
- Proteins
- Calcium
  and
- Complexity of carbohydrates

- *Avocados*

According to the *U.S. Department of Agriculture,* avocados offer us, inter alia,

- Vitamin B/E/K
  as well as
- Healthy fats

Additionally, they are an excellent source of 'good'

- HDL cholesterol

based on research at, inter alia, *Tufts University* in Boston, MA.

Not to overlook the power of colored avocado seed extracts may fight colon/breast/prostate cancer cells

Based on research at, inter alia, *Pennsylvania State University* at University Park, PA.

Fruits

- *Apples*

You may know the saying "An apple a day keeps the doctor away."

At least, according to research at *Cornell University* in Ithaca, NY, and the *University of Alaska* in Fairbanks, AK, apples may cut down risk of chronic disease and extend life span.

- *Blueberries*

According to research in Germany, at the *Technical University of Munich* and *Albstadt-Sigmaringen University* in Sigmaringen, blueberries not only may not only help against cognitive decline and Alzheimer's but also may help to prevent cardiovascular disease.

Also, based on research at *Shenyang Agricultural University* in Shenyang, China, blueberries may reduce obesity.

Not to forget that, according to clinical trial by the *Grady Health System* in Atlanta, GA, blueberries may cut blood pressure stage 1 in females.

Nuts

- *Almonds*

are certainly one of the most nutritious foods because of their content of

- Vitamin E
- Calcium
- Magnesium
- Fiber
- Iron
and

- Riboflavin

with the special benefit of reducing total cholesterol.

According to research at, inter alia, *Tufts University* in Boston, MA.

- *Brazil nuts*

is an excellent source of

- Vitamins B-1 & E
- Selenium
- Magnesium
- Zinc
- Proteins
  and
- Carbohydrates

And therefore beneficial to support our thyroid function.

According to, inter alia, the U.S. *National Institutes of Health.*

Oatmeal

Based on comprehensive research in Taiwan at, inter alia

- *National Taiwan University* in Taipei
- *National Yang-Ming University* in Taipei
- *National Taiwan University College of Medicine and Hospital* in Taipei
- *Taipei Veterans General Hospital* in Taipei
- *Mackay Medical College* in New Taipei City
- *Tzu-Chi University* in Hualien
- *China Medical University Hospital* in Taichung
- *Kaohsiung Medical University* in Kaohsiung
- *Far Eastern Memorial Hospital* in New Taipei City
- *E-Da Hospital* (Kaohsiung, Taiwan)

oatmeal – with its high fiber content - may not only lower cholesterol but also cut down cardiovascular risk factors in general.

Lentils

This pulse, rich in

- Fiber
- Potassium
- Selenium
- Magnesium
- Folic acid

helping, inter alia, with

- heart health

   by reducing cholesterol and high blood pressure, with its folic acid and potassium according to research at, inter alia, *Johns Hopkins Bloomberg School of Public Health* in Baltimore, MD, and the *University of Minnesota School of Public Health* in Minneapolis, MN

   Also in cases of

- pregnancy

   to prevent neural tube defects with its folic acid according to *Harvard T.H. Chan School of Public Health* in Boston, MA, and *Statens Serum Institut* in Copenhagen, Denmark

And for

- cancer

   to reduce tumor growth with selenium according to *Universitas Andalas* in Padang City and *Universitas Gadjah Mada* in Yogyakarta City – both Indonesia.

Fish

When talking about fish, it is primarily *oily* fish like

- salmon
- mackerel
- trout
- sardines
- herring
  and
- anchovies

containing high amounts of *omega-3 fatty acids* as well as vitamins A & D.

With the health benefits for, inter alia, our heart, nervous system and rheumatoid arthritis.

According to research at, inter alia, the *Karolinska Institutet* in Stockholm, Sweden.

Chicken

Primarily free-range chicken because of their content of protein with special reference to their 'posterity' – the eggs.

These are not only an excellent source of protein as well but also of vitamins B-2 & B-12.

CONTRAST

Unfortunately yet, the major part of our population in modern times subsists in terms of taste and satiety with non-healthy diet.

With the result that, according to the *World Health Organization (WHO)* in our industrialized societies
- 86% of non-age-related deaths
  and
- 77% of all ailments combined

are the consequence of 'chronic' health issues. With special reference to, inter alia, heart failure, hypertension, diabetes 2, depression and cancer, etc.

Primarily due to manufactured/ultra-processed foods and added sugars which contain no or not enough whole foods. With the seemingly only benefit for the consumer to be convenient and imperishable.

Scientifically validated only recently by, inter alia, the *University of Navarra* in Pamplona, Spain.

IN A NUTSHELL

Nature gives us unlimited access to appropriate diet for health and longevity. In this chapter you experience a brief excursion to consider. Without being/becoming vegetarian or vegan.

10. SUPPORT YOUR HEALTH WITH PLANTAINS

THE PHILOSOPHY BEHIND

To live a long and healthy life, your body and mind needs healthy diet, since man has entered our globe the Earth millions of years ago. Including nutritious fruits we find plenty in nature's kingdom.

One of these highly valuable fruits are *plantains* (biologic name: *musa x paradisiaca*), a special type of bananas as a rich source of vitamins (A/B-6/C) and minerals (magnesium/potassium), as well as proteins, antioxidants and fiber. According to the U.S. Department of Agriculture.

Native primarily to Africa, Asia, parts of Latin America and the West Indies, but available also in our northern hemisphere.

Usually to be cooked (baked/boiled/fried/etc.) in different stages of ripeness (i.e. when it is green/yellow/black) before eaten. Including the dried and grinded flour of green plantains to be consumed in the Caribbean and West Indian cooking.

HEALTH BENEFITS = SCIENTIFICALLY VERIFIED

According to research at, inter alia, *Harvard T.H. Chan School of Public Health* in Boston, MA, the inherent *fiber* compound helps with, inter alia,
- Diabetes
- Heart disease
- Constipation
- Diverticular disease

Also, the *antioxidants polyphenols* and *flavonoids* fight free radicals known to cause oxidative stress damaging our body.

Based on research at, inter alia, the *University of Fort Hare* in Alice, South Africa, and the *National Institute for Interdisciplinary Science and Technology* in Thiruvananthapuram, India.

No less important its anti-inflammatory power and the support for a stronger immune system with plantains' inherent *vitamins A* and *C*.

According to research at, inter alia, *Penn State University* in Hershey, PA, and *Guilin Medical University* in Guangxi, China.

Not to overlook plantains' powerful *potassium* content to cut down per se, and the risk of high blood pressure.

Based on research at, inter alia,
- *Harvard Medical School* in Boston, MA
- *Beni-Suef University* in Beni-Suef, Egypt
and
- *Imam Abdulrahman Bin Fasal University* in Dammam, Saudi Arabia.

As well as the strength of inherent *vitamin B-6* not only is good for heart and mind, along with *magnesium* it may also help with depression and anxiety. According to research at, inter alia, the *University of Massachusetts* in Lowell, MA, and *Tufts University* in Boston's suburbia Medford/Somerville, MA.

IN A NUTSHELL

Plantains are a type of bananas native to Africa, Asia, Latin America and the West Indies - but available also on our markets in the northern hemisphere. With quite a few highly nutritious components for our health, as focused on in this chapter, which you may not want to miss.

11. WEIGHT LOSS OR WEIGHT MANAGEMENT?

THE PHILOSOPHY BEHIND

Lacking appropriate body weight is one of the leading health issues in the industrialized world. With two thirds of the adult population in the industrialized world being overweight, and half of those even obese, i.e. at least 30% beyond of what it got to be. With severe consequences for health, with special reference to cardiovascular events and all-case mortality.

However, even if you understand how important weight loss may well be for your health and longevity in general, you may still run in circles as the victim of *malnutrition*.

Not to be understood in this case in terms of not enough food – but lack of right nutrients, and at the right time.

As clearly indicated by recent research at the *University Hospital Alvaro Cunqueiro* in Vigo, Spain. Scientifically verified also at, inter alia, the *University of Florida* in Gainesville, FL, and the *National Jewish Health* hospital in Denver, CO.

WEIGHT MANAGEMENT – SCIENTIFICALLY VERIFIED

Fortunately, there are ways to *manage* our weight with respect to quantity, quality and organization of our diet, in line with nature.

Inter alia,

Healthy diet

In line with recommendations of the *American Heart Association (AHA),* healthy diet should be made up as follows:
- 50% fruits and vegetables
- 25% whole grains (including brown rice and oatmeal) and
- 25% protein

Surrounded by
- 25-30 grams (g) of fiber daily.

Vice-versa, avoid
- fatty red meat

- processed foods
- foods with added oils/butter/sugar
- baked goods
- white bread
- bagels

Mindful Eating

Mindful eating is more than just 'grab a bite' where and whenever you can. Rather, it is conscious handling for the best of your health.

Based on research at, inter alia, the *University of California* in San Francisco.

E.g.,

- Choose wisely

food you not only like but which is healthy with the appropriate nutrients at the same time.

The U.S. *Centers for Disease Control and Prevention (CDC)* recommend plenty of vegetables, fruits and whole grain. And only low dairy products. Proteins only from lean meats, poultry, fish, eggs and nuts.

At the same time, the CDC discourages of eating much of

- cholesterol containing food
- trans and saturated fats
- large amounts of sugar and salt

- Eat slowly

in order to give your brain the chance telling you when 'enough is enough', to avoid over-eating – and overweight.

- Take time

sitting down, without distraction by watching TV or driving a car at the same time, etc.

Intermitting Fasting

Short-term fasting at regular times during the day up to half a year can well initiate weight loss. With following options:

- Alternate Day Fasting (ADF)

i.e. eat regular (health food) only every second day.

- 5:2 Diet

with no food restrictions 5 days of the week and 400-500 calories less on the remaining 2 days.

- 16/8 Fasting

I.e. .limit eating to only 8 hours per day.

- Whole day Fasting

at certain days of the week
with 2

- Time restricted feeding

to eat at a certain time frame (e.g. between 8 a,m, and 3 p.m.) and fasting during remaining hours of day

Aocording to research at, inter alia,
- *Queen Mary's School of Medicine* in London, UK
- *University Hospital of South Manchester,* UK
- *Aarhus University Hospital* in Aarhus, Denmark
- *Harvard T. Chan School of Public Health* in Boston, MA
- *National Clinical Guideline Center* (hosted by the *Royal College of Physicians*) in London, UK

Based on this research is also the recommendation for

Low calorie meal plan

as follows.

- Breakfast

- one medium size slice of whole wheat bread with 2 teaspoons (tsp) jelly
- ¾ cup of orange juice
- ½ cup of shredded wheat with 1 cup of milk
- 1 cup regular coffee
- adding proteins to your breakfast (in form of e.g. eggs, quinoa,

sardines, oats, porridge, chia seed pudding, etc.) is rising the hormonal satiety effect, avoiding over-eating already in the morning.

- Lunch

  - Roast beef sandwich with 2 medium slices whole wheat bread, 2 ounces (oz) of lean/unseasoned roast beef, 1 lettuce leaf, 3 slices of tomato, and 1 tsp low calorie mayonnaise
  - 1 medium apple
  - 1 cup of water

- Dinner

  - ½ cup of green beans
  - 1 small white dinner roll
  - ¾ medium baked potato with 1 tsp mayonnaise on top
  - 2 oz salmon cooked in 1.5 tsp vegetable oil
  - ½ cup carrots
  - 1 cup unsweetened iced tea
  - 2 cups of water

IN A NUTSHELL

Two thirds of the adult population in the industrialized world are overweight, and half of those even obese. With severe consequences for health and longevity. However, cutting down the quantity of food is not enough, focusing on its quality and organization of our diet is equally important.

12. FIGHT INFECTION WITH YOUR IMMUNITY

THE PHILOSOPHY BEHIND

Our physical and mental existence is a perfect biologic-ecologic phenomenon. Centrally supported by our inherent natural immune system.

This implies that we need to maintain our immune system (in line with the natural self-healing power of our body) to ward off diseases. Yes, with special reference to *infections*.

However, as we age also our immune system is losing ground. I.e., not only does it become weaker, it also becomes imbalanced.

Associated with chronic inflammation, leading the way to most health issues we are facing later in life. infection being no exception. As scientifically verified at, inter alia, *Soochow University Medical College* in Suzhou and *Shanghai Institutes for Biological Sciences* in Shanghai, both China.

This refers to *innate* and *adaptive* immunity alike.

Innate Immunity

Innate immunity being our first line of defense against infections which is failing to resolve when initial threat has passed, leading to kind of chronic/systemic inflammation.

According to research at, inter alia, *Queen's University Belfast* in Belfast, the *University College Dublin* in Dublin and the *University of Ulster* in Londonderry – all 3 UK – as well as *Mayo Clinic* in Jacksonville, Florida.

This is especially true for elder people who therefore are more prone for, inter alia, cardiovascular disease, cancer, diabetes 2 and neurodegenerative ailments and other typically age-related health issues. That's why we are talking about 'inflammaging'.

Supported by research at, inter alia, the

- *Sigmund Freud Private University* in Austria's capital Vienna,
- *University of Giessen* in Giessen, Germany
  and in Japan at the

- *University of Toyama* in Toyama,
- *Hokkaido University Graduate School of Medicine* in Sapporo, and
- *Sapporo Asabu Neurosurgical Hospital* in Sapporo as well.

Adaptive Immunity

On the other hand, adaptive immunity helping our body to remember and attack pathogens, loses its power with progressive age to defend us against bacteria, viruses, and fungi, and also can reactivate pathogens previously suppressed. With the additional negative consequence that a weakened adaptive immunity later in life may give less strength to help with vaccinations, flu shots included.

According to research at, inter alia, the *University of Chicago* in Chicago, IL, and the *University of Tübingen* in Tübingen, Germany.

SUPPORT IMMUNITY NATURALLY – SCIENTIFICALLY VERIFIED

In order to keep our immune system intact even later in life to ward off infections and other health issues, we can adjust our lifestyle accordingly. With special reference to physical activity and healthy diet. Scientifically validated internationally.

Physical Activity

According to research at, inter alia, the
- *University of Birmingham* in Birmingham, UK
- *University of Houston* in Houston, TX
- *Edinburgh Napier University* in Edinburgh, UK
- *University of Freiburg* in Freiburg, Germany
  and the
- *University of Sao Paulo* in Sao Paulo, Brazil

physical exercise is not only of high relevance for our immune system per se, but for seniors in particular.

While there are quite a few different physical activities to consider, just pick the 4 most beneficial.

- **Running**

Although it got to be practiced over some weeks or even months – usually free of charge and without certain equipment or specific training – in your neighborhood, wherever it is. Starting with a couple of minutes to extend the time according to feasibility and fun.

Similar effect comes with

- ***Walking***

Although it is of lower intensity than running, there are advantages. Because not only is it easier to move ahead longer stretches of way than with running but this can be performed in any environment, e.g. in the countryside and/or on the beach, etc., with potentially more motivation and enjoyment.

- ***Cycling***

is even more intense than walking because of the higher leg performance, especially by pushing pedals faster and uphill. Regardless if cycling to and from work regularly, or just for fun.

- ***Swimming***

This form of exercise is one of the best for losing calories. Although it may not be that handy like walking, if you do not live on poolside ore close to woods or shore.

Healthy Diet

While healthy diet is of general importance for our health, vitamin D and polyunsaturated acids (as part of, inter alia, Mediterranean diet) are especially important to ward off infections and frailty because of their anti-inflammatory properties.

According to research at, inter alia, the *University College London*, UK

With special reference to the fact that seniors tend to weight gain with 'inflammaging', according to research at, inter alia, *Sorbonne University* in Paris, France, and therefore may be prone to catching infections.

As a brief collection, these are the nutrients of Mediterranean diet supporting the immune system, as recommended and validated, inter alia, by the *American Heart Association:*

- High volume of vegetables and fruits
- Nuts and seeds
- High fiber starches like beans, potatoes, whole grain bread, etc.
- Poultry and fish
- Eggs up to 4 times a week

IN A NUTSHELL

As central part of our biologic-ecologic existence, our immune system can ward off health issues. With special reference also to viral infections and related inflammation. While this power of our immune system is weakening and becoming imbalanced later in life, we can counteract naturally with physical exercise and healthy diet.

13. WHICH FOODS TO SAVE YOUR HEART?

THE PHILOSOPHY BEHIND

According to the World Health Organization (WHO), 86% of non-age-related premature deaths in our industrialized countries are the result of debilitating non-solved health issues. With heart failure on top of the list (followed by cancer). Basically due to self-applied unfavorable lifestyle factors. With poor physical activity and unhealthy diet leading this pattern. The latter due to lack of sufficient health food, manifold replaced by unhealthy processed food. This leaves us with the question about ...

HEALTH FOOD FOR OUR HEART – SCIENTIFICALLY VALIDATED

Nature's kingdom is brimming unlimited with food supporting for our health and longevity generally, and for heart health specifically. Tapped by our ancestors with enthusiasm for thousands of years. Although this health food is still available – for free and at low cost at least – wherever we live, our knowledge about has shrunk in our seemingly 'modern' times.

That's why we are focusing in this blog on at least a small part of heart healthy nutrition. Based on recommendations of the U.S. governmental *Centers for Disease Control and Prevention (CDC)* and scientifically verified internationally.

In more detail:

- ***Broccoli***

This cruciferous green leafy vegetable may prevent heart disease by lowering artery-blocking cholesterol in blood.

According to research at, inter alia, *Vanderbilt University School of Medicine* in Nashville, TN. Scientifically verified also at the *Western Regional Research Center* of USDA-ARS in Albany, New York.

Similar

- ***Legumes/pulses***

like peas/lentils/beans/chickpeas not only can lower the heart-harming LDL cholesterol, their contents of, inter alia, protein, fiber and antioxidant polyphenols are beneficial for health in general and heart health in particular.

Based on research at, inter alia, the *University of Toronto* and *St. Michael's Hospital,* both in Toronto, Canada.

In this context we may also see

- ***Oatmeal***

Because of its high content of soluble fiber to cut down 'bad' LDL cholesterol considerably.

According to research at, inter alia, the *University of Kentucky* in Lexington, KY.

- ***Spinach***

As it is an excellent source of magnesium, spinach helps with healthy heart rhythm and other heart benefits.

With reference to research at, inter alia, the *Linus Pauling Institute* at *Oregon State University* in Corvallis, OR.

- ***Tomatoes***

are heart healthy too because of highly powerful nutrients like primarily potassium but also because of its content of vitamin C, choline and folate (vitamin B-9).

According to, inter alia, the U.S. governmental *Centers for Disease Control and Prevention* in Atlanta, GA.

Besides of potassium's benefits also for muscle strength and bones, as well as it may prevent kidney stones.

- ***Asparagus***

Since it contains folate preventing to build up the amino acid homocysteine, it helps to ward off coronary artery disease (CAD) and stroke.

Based on research at, inter alia, *Alfaisal University,* as well as the *King Faisal Specialized Hospital and Research Centre* – both in Riyadh, Saudi Arabia.

- ***Nuts***

As nuts (like peanuts/pistachios/almonds/pecans/hazelnuts/walnuts) are rich in vitamins/minerals/fiber/protein/antioxidants, and especially walnuts being ripe with omega-3 fatty acids, they are very heart-healthy.

According to, inter alia, the *American Heart Association.*

- ***Green tea***

This beverage is not only delicious but beneficial for our health – especially our heart.

By reducing 'bad' LDL cholesterol, based on research at, inter alia, *University of Connecticut School of Pharmacy* in Hartford, CT.

And cutting down high blood pressure, according to, inter alia, *Griffith University* in Gold Coast, Australia.

- ***Flaxseed /Chia seeds***

Similar to also chia seeds, flaxseed is rich in omega-3 fatty acids like alpha-linoleic acid which lowers total cholesterol – especially LDL. Reducing high blood pressure, accordingly.

Since omega-3 is also cutting down the risk of arrhythmias and thrombosis known to potentially leading to heart attack.

Based on research at, inter alia, the *University of Manitoba* and *St. Boniface General Hospital* – both in in Winnipeg, Canada – and *VI Lenin University Hospital* in Holguin, Cuba.

In this context we may also appreciate

- ***Fish***

As a most valuable source of omega-3 fatty acids (and protein) lowering the risk of abnormal heartbeat.

Verified by the *American Heart Association.*

- ***Berries***

This fruit is highly valuable for our cardiovascular health in general. Based on its content of, inter alia, vitamins (A/B-9/C), minerals (calcium & iron), as well as fiber.

Based on research at, inter alia, *Oklahoma State University* in Stillwater, OK.

- ***Liver***

Liver is very important for our heart health, as it is a most nutrient-dense organ meat with special reference to minerals copper/zinc/iron/chromium, and folic acid.

According to research at, inter alia, *Linus Pauling Institute* at *Oregon State University* in Corvallis, OR.

- ***Dark Chocolate***

does not only fondle our taste buds, it helps against atherosclerosis (buildup of plaque in our arteries potentially leading to heart attack and stroke).

According to research at, inter alia, *Wageningen University* in Wageningen, The Netherlands.

IN A NUTSHELL

According to World Health Organization (WHO) statistics, heart disease is the # 1 of non-age-related premature deaths in the industrialized world. The cause: lack of physical activity and unhealthy diet. In this chapter we focused on a sample of natural food supporting your heart naturally. Scientifically validated. Inter alia, by the Linus Pauling Institute at Oregon State University, founded by U.S. Nobel Prize Laureate Dr. Linus Pauling.

14. SAVE YOUR HEALTH WITH NATURE!

THE PHILOSOPHY BEHIND

Needless to stress that good health is the basic prerequisite for a long and happy life. Although healthcare costs in the U.S. are more than $3.5 trillion (!) per year, according to the governmental *Centers for Disease Control and Prevention (CDC),* this country ranks at position 31 on World Health Organization (WHO) list of international life expectancy only.

Therefore, it is important to follow up and understand what *health* is all about to support and materialize the goal of good health at least personally.

COMPLEXITY OF HEALTH – SCIENTIFICALLY VALIDATED

In fact, health is not a singular issue of physical well-being, but a complexity of health issues, just as WHO put it straight already more than 70 years ago in its constitution:

"Health is a state of complete physical, mental and social well-being and not merely the absence of disease or infirmity."

With physical and mental issues in the forefront, complemented also by spiritual, emotional and financial health.

Besides of potential

- genetic factors

which may well play a role in health. At least in cases of an unusual genetic pattern or if specific inherited genes may lead to certain health conditions.

Also

- environmental factors

do play a role with respect to health. In terms of
- social and economic environment (e.g. low socio-economic status leading to stress-related health issues, etc.)
  and
- physical environment (e.g. pollution, etc.)

Just as

- cultural factors

can have an impact on health with customs and traditions of a certain society.

To make a long story short, let's focus on physical and mental health criteria in following.

Physical health

Physical health, however, is not only the absence of disease. Rather, it is a complexity of vital issues like

- *Regular exercise*

to maintain physical fitness supporting, inter alia,
- Heart function
- Breathing
- Muscle strength
and also reducing risk of injuries and health issues.

- *Balanced nutrition*
  with, minerals, vitamins, fiber, proteins, carbohydrates, fat and water involved.

In this context, when following a *Mediterranean* diet with lots of whole grain, olive oil, fruits and vegetables, this may give you a lower 10-year all-cause mortality rate. According to research at, inter alia, the *University of Medicine and Pharmacy* and *Sf. Spiridon Emergency Hospital* – both in Iasi, Romania.

As well as

- *Adequate rest with sound sleep at night*

Thereby, physical health is strongly related to

Mental health

According to the U.S. Department of Health & Human Services, this is with reference to
- emotional
- psychological

and
-    social
well-being.

This is no less important than physical health – although manifold overlooked.

Not only in cases of depression, anxiety or anorexia which may enhance the risk of health disorders.

Based on research at, inter alia, the *Veteran Affairs Medical Center* in Tuscaloosa, AL.

Especially, as good mental health is also strongly related to the ability of
-    enjoying life
-    feeling safe and secure
-    handling bad experiences (e.g. family issues or finances) and adapting to better alternatives

Accordingly, it is important to see the close and complex relationship between physical and mental health instead of a series of different and seemingly independent factors only.

POTENTIAL LIMITATIONS

You may, however, face some kind of 'unhappiness' when evaluating your health. E.g., if you are obliged to partial or complete 'lockdown' with stay-at-home orders, as this may require, and lead to, unhealthful changes.

Such as lack of physical activities due to sedentary lifestyle, and mentally in terms of anxiety or depression involved.

According to research at, inter alia, *Louisiana State University*'s Pennington Biomedical Research Center in Baton Rouge, LA.

IN A NUTSHELL

Good health is the basic prerequisite for long and happy life. Unfortunately yet, the U.S. ranks low in terms of life expectancy internationally. Despite of highest costs p.c. in health care in the industrialized world, summing up to $3.5 trillion per year. This chapter may show you how to support and materialize the goal of good health, naturally. Scientifically validated.

15. CAUGHT A COLD? RELEASE WITH NATURE!

THE PHILOSOPHY BEHIND

Many of us may suffer physically and/or mentally from pandemic these days. Overlooking a wintery relative, well known since time immemorial and still on the horizon: the common cold. Fortunately, nature got powerful answers in this case we may not want to underestimate.

FIGHT COLD WITH HERBS – SCIENTIFICALLY VERIFIED

While nature's kingdom got an almost unlimited portfolio of powerful herbs to fight the cold, let's focus on following selection. Appreciated by our ancestors for their health as a tea since thousands of years - and scientifically validated internationally today. (See scientific botanical names in brackets.)

Chamomile
(Matricaria chamomilla)

Known from experience over millennia, chamomile may support our immune system and fight infections triggering common cold.

Validated scientifically by, inter alia,
- *Case Western Reserve University*
- *University Hospitals Case Medical Center*
  and
- *Case Comprehensive Cancer Center*
all in Cleveland, Ohio.

Echinacea
(Echinacea purpurea)

This herb is widely used for common cold in North America and Europe.

According to research at, inter alia, the
- *University of Arizona* in Tucson, Arizona,
- *University of Wisconsin* in Madison, Wisconsin
  as well as at the
- *Technical University of Munich*, Germany
  and the
- *Karl-Franzens University* in Graz, Austria

Ginger
(Zingiber officinale)

may help in cases of common cold with, inter alia, congestion problems and sore throat.

Scientifically verified at, inter alia, *Dalhousie University* at Canadian campuses of Halifax and Truro. As well as the *Chinese Academy of Agricultural Sciences* in China's capital Beijing.

Elderberry
(Sambucus nigra L.)

To help mitigating respiratory symptoms and cutting down duration of the cold. As well as it may serve against inflammation and as an antioxidant for our immune system.

Based on research at, inter alia,
- *University of Waterloo* in Waterloo, Canada
  and
- *Poznan University of Life Sciences* in Poznan, Poland

Peppermint
(Mentha x piperita)

Known to support the immune system, reduce cell mutation and improve cardiovascular health while fighting the cold.

Also, the menthol in peppermint may relieve clogged sinuses for better breathing.

According to research at, inter alia,
- *Kermanshah University of Medical Sciences* in Kermanshah, Iran
  and the
- *National Institute of Genetic Engineering and Biotechnology* in Iran's capital Tehran

Not to forget about

Green tea
(Camellia sinensis)

Besides other benefits for our health, it has a reputation to reduce coughing, also in cases of common cold.

Scientifically verified by research at, inter alia

- *Kyoto University* in Kyoto
  and the
- *University of Shizuoka* in Shizuoka
both in Japan

IN A NUTSHELL

Currently buffeted physically/mentally by the wind of viral infections worldwide, we may not forget about a relative of this pandemic, well-known since generations: the common cold. Fortunately, nature got a portfolio of medicinal herbs to help with. In this blog we focus on some of those – scientifically validated.

16. NATURE'S MAGIC ANSWER FOR DEPRESSION

THE PHILOSOPHY BEHIND

Based on statistics of the U.S. *National Institute of Mental Health,* more than 17 million adults have at least one depressive episode in life. As the most debilitating mental health issue in this country. Mostly treated with addictive anti-depressant drugs – the 3rd most prescribed drugs (after painkillers and cholesterol statins). Raising the premature, i.e. non-age-related death risk by one third.

With special reference to some 70 most dangerous long-term side effects. Such as, inter alia,
- Bleeding in brain
(according to research at, inter alia, *Western University* in London, Canada)
- Thickening of arteries as a potential cause of heart attack and stroke
(based on research at, inter alia, *Emory University School of Medicine* in Druid Hills, GA, and the *University of Queensland* in Brisbane, Australia)
Not to forget about potential
- Birth defects
(as scientifically validated by the U.S. governmental *Centers for Disease Control and Prevention (CDC).*

As you have learned already from our previous publications, there are quite a few natural remedies to relieve depression such as, inter alia, vitamins B-9 (folic acid), B-12, and vitamin D. Additionally to members of nature's kingdom of herbs such as ashwagandha, roseroot, magnolia, black cohosh and St. John's wort. Verified by U.S. and international research.

Now we learn also about

NATURE'S >MAGIC MUSHROOM< – SCIENTIFICALLY VERIFIED

when it comes to powerful relief of depression.

Due to the antidepressant property of its constituent *psilocybin.*

Based on research at, inter alia, *Johns Hopkins University* in Baltimore, MD, the *University of Paris XII* in Creteil, France, and *Palo Alto*

University in Palo Alto, CA, according to which the antidepressant effect may last even 5 years, dropping severity in more than 70% of cases.

IN A NUTSHELL

Depression is one of the most debilitating mental health issues in our industrialized world. Manifold treated with the 3rd most prescribed drugs (after painkillers and cholesterol statins) with some 70 side effects - raising premature death risk by one third. Now you have learned in this chapter about a 'magic' and highly potent natural remedy for relief. Validated by U.S. and international medical research.

17. DROP HIGH BLOOD PRESSURE DRUG-FREE

THE PHILOSOPHY BEHIND

The term blood pressure indicates the force of the heart pumping blood through the whole body. Pushing the blood against artery walls made up of the relationship between 'systolic' pressure (upper value, when the heart beats) and 'diastolic' pressure (lower value, between heartbeats). Expressed by millimeters of mercury (mm Hg).

When this force becomes higher than 120 mm Hg/systolic (and higher than 80 mm Hg diastolic), we speak about high blood pressure ('hypertension'), according to the American Heart Association in Dallas, TX, and the *American College of Cardiology* in Washington, D.C. Increasing the risk of coronary heart disease by at least 50% and of stroke by more than 70%.

According to statistics of U.S. governmental Centers for Disease Control and Prevention, some 75 million U.S. citizens. i.e. more than 30% of adults have high blood pressure.

Killing more than 600,000 U.S. citizens with heart disease per year - # 1 cause of non-age-related cause of death.

In fact, based on research at, inter alia, the *University of California and Kaiser Permanente Medical Center* (both Los Angeles, CA), and the *Universitätsklinikum Erlangen* in Erlangen, Germany, high blood pressure has very high impact on the cardiovascular system.

Such as, inter alia
- heart failure
  (failure of heart to pump enough blood due to increase of pressure on vessels)
- heart attack
  (blocked flow of oxygen-rich blood to part of the heart)
- angina
- stroke
- blood clots
- aneurysm
  (abnormal bulge in blood vessel wall leading, inter alia, to pressure on other organs, blocking flood flow and even burst)
- memory problems

To avoid this vicious cycle, it is indispensable to manage your heart pressure, especially if it is already too high.

For this purpose, you got 2 opportunities: synthetic drugs (with debilitating side effects involved, extending the vicious cycle). And

NATURE'S ANSWERS – SCIENTIFICALLY VALIDATED

While these natural answers are almost unlimited, let's focus on a couple of powerful natural opportunities with special reference to easily adjustable (and inexpensive) lifestyle and nutritional factors. Verified by the American Heart Association.

Physical exercise

Exercising regularly not only makes your heart stronger and more efficient for pumping blood. It also reduces high blood pressure
According to research at, inter alia,
- *University of Louisville* in Louisville, KY
- *University of Michigan* in Ann Arbor, MI
- *University of South Carolina* in Columbia, SC
- *University of Costa Rica in San Jose*, Costa Rica
and
- *Inje University College of Medicine* in Busan, South Korea

With special reference to aerobic activity of
- 150 minutes of moderate exercise (walking)
    or
- 75-150 minutes vigorous exercise (running)
as based on research at the *Catholic University of Leuven* in Leuven, Belgium, and the *University of New England* in Armidale, Australia.

According to research at the *University of California* in San Francisco, CA, for every 1,000 steps walking per day, blood pressure may be approximately lower by 0.45 points.

Weight management

Already losing 5% of weight can reduce blood pressure considerably. According to *Texas A&M University* in Dallas, TX.

Weight loss of 1 kilogram (2.2 pounds) may lower blood pressure by around 1 mm/HG, according to the American College of Cardiology and the American Heart Association.

Losing more than 17 pounds (approx. 8 kg) of weight may lower systolic blood pressure by 8.5 mm and diastolic blood pressure by 6.5 mm Hg. Based on research at *Duke University Medical Center* in Durham, NC.

Healthy diet

Healthy diet, besides physical exercise, is one of the 2 basic pillars our life expectancy stands on. Basically, nature's kingdom of nutrition is unlimited in this respect, with special reference to support of appropriate blood pressure. As verified by the American Heart Association.

Just take foods rich in following minerals as a small example.

The mineral

- Magnesium

is most helpful to control blood pressure, supporting our immune system and many functions in our body.

Based on medical research at, inter alia, *Stanford University* in Stanford, California, *Indiana University in Bloomington*, Indiana, *McGill University* in Montreal, Canada, and *Fukushima Medical University* in Fukushima, Japan.

You find magnesium in whole nutrition such as, inter alia,

- Black beans
- Brown rice
- Cashews
- Peanuts

- Calcium

is another highly potent mineral to cut down high blood pressure, based on research at, inter alia, *Aga Khan University* in Karachi, Pakistan. To be found in, inter alia,

- Spinach
- Almonds
- Avocados
- Low-fat/fat-free yogurt

In fact, according to research at, inter alia, *Emory University* in Atlanta, GA, both minerals – magnesium and calcium – have the power to decrease high blood pressure. With special reference to the fact that both minerals counteract heart-harming sodium. Scientifically verified also by the *University of Virginia* in Charlottesville, VA.

Unfortunately yet, many Americans live in areas where magnesium and calcium is short in drinking water. Especially as groundwater is main source of drinking water for those living in coastal regions.

That's why fortification of drinking water with these minerals may well be beneficial.

Also, we may not overlook the importance of

- Potassium

which is equally helpful. Balancing out excess salt derived from unhealthy diet which otherwise hinders kidneys getting rid of excess water from the body, thus increasing blood pressure. As it reduces the effect of salt/sodium and also the tension in blood vessel walls, accordingly.
The American Heart Association recommends a daily consumption of 4,700 milligrams (mg) of potassium per day.

You find this powerful nutrient in

- Tomatoes
- Sweet & regular potatoes
- Leafy greens
- Spinach
- Mushrooms
- Nuts/seeds
- Beans
- Melons
- Bananas
- Oranges
- Apricots
- Low-fat/fat-free yogurt
- Milk
- Avocados
- Prunes
- Tuna
- Etc.

Based on research at, inter alia, *Emory University* in Atlanta, GA, the *University of Southern California* in Los Angeles, CA, *Harvard School of Public Health* in Boston, MA, and the *University of Modena* in Modena, Italy.

Stress reduction

Stress is certainly a basic parameter for raising blood pressure, with faster heart rate and constricted blood vessels involved.
In order to relieve, you may, inter alia,

- listen to soothing music

for relaxation of your nervous system.
Based on research at, inter alia, the *M.S. Ramaiah Medical College* and the *Gokula Education Foundation* – both in Bangalore, India – as well as the *Federal University of Sergipe* in Sao Cristovao, Brazil.

Also

- less (especially stressful) work

may cut down blood pressure.

According to research at, inter alia, *Nantong University* in Nantong and *Xinjiang Medical University* in Urumqi – both China – and the *University of California* in Irvine, CA.

Sound sleep

Based on research at *Pusan National University School of Medicine* and *Pusan National University Hospital* – both in Pusan, South Korea – people with less than 5 hours of sleep per night are endangered health wise.

To benefit our blood pressure, nighttime sleep should not be less than 6 hours according to research at, inter alia, the *Pennsylvania State College of Medicine* in Hershey, PA.

Based on research at *Columbia University Irving Medical Center* in New York, even mild sleep problems may initiate vascular endothelial inflammation with negative consequence for our cardiovascular system with special reference to blood pressure and heart attack, especially for females.

Quit smoking

Finally for those who (still) smoke:

Chemicals in tobacco increase blood pressure and damage blood vessels, based on research at, inter alia, *Mt. Sinai School of Medicine* in New York, NY.

IN A NUTSHELL

High blood pressure (hypertension) is related to greatest contradiction in our life. On one side, it may look harmless, as it is not painful; on the other,

It is the #1 cause behind premature and non-age-related deaths in our 'civilized' society. Not enough. Many of those diagnosed with hypertension swallow drugs with considerable side effects to suppress the mmHg numbers without tackling the real cause behind. Fortunately, nature got right answers for powerful and drug-free blood pressure management.

18. HOW MANAGE ECZEMA NATURALLY

THE PHILOSOPHY BEHIND

Some 10% of the U.S. population – independent of age/race/gender/etc. – are hit by eczema leading to itchy and dry skin and sometimes swelling and infections. If you are one of those, you don't have to tackle it with chemical synthetics causing additional health issues and without solving the problem.

Rather, trust nature with its 'kingdom' of natural remedies and modalities for any health issue – eczema being no exception.

In order to downsize this natural inventory, just see a small selection of

NATURAL ANSWERS – SCIENTIFICALLY VALIDATED

in terms of remedies and modalities as follows. To fight, relieve and avoid dryness, itching and infection of the skin. Easily applicable and economically affordable. Scientifically verified and recommended by the U.S. National Eczema Association (NEA).

Not only as an application not only on the outside of the body - the skin - but also internally as a physiological exchange. Based on the fact that any living species on this planet is a complex biologic-ecologic phenomenon strictly based on natural laws – man included.

Just let us start with ...

Honey

which is antibacterial and anti-inflammatory to prevent and fight infections.

Therefore honey is recommended scientifically to tackle eczema with it according to research at, inter alia, *Nazarbayev University* in Astana, Kazakhstan, *Neyshabur University of Medical Sciences* in Neyshabur, Iran, and *Queen Margaret University* in Edinburgh, UK.

Apple Cider Vinegar

is just one other of those recommendations, with special reference to its antimicrobial activity, according to research at, inter alia, *Middlesex University* in London, UK, to fight respective bacteria involved.

To be used diluted (only) – to avoid burns at same time – in baths (15-20 minutes) or with wet wraps (3 hours).

Also

Virgin Coconut Oil

helps if pressed cold on the eczema several times a day to add moisture to the skin with the fatty acids it contains to avoid skin dryness.

Based on research at, inter alia, the *Jose R. Reyes Memorial Medical Center* in Manila, Philippines.

Tea Tree Oil

is not only antibacterial, anti-inflammatory, wound healing and preventing infections but also may relieve itching and dryness of the skin.

Before applying, dilute this essential oil and mix it with a carrier oil like olive oil.

According to research at, inter alia, *Ahvaz Iidishapur University of Medical Sciences* in Ahvaz, Iran.

Since eczema is inflaming the skin, research at, inter alia, *Baylor College of Medicine* in Houston, TX, recommends

Nutritional Factors

with anti-inflammatory power such as

- colorful fruits
- vegetables/leafy greens
- beans/lentils
- fish

to avoid eczema flares.

Along with anti-inflammatory

Herbs

such as cinnamon and turmeric.

Turmeric has been already documented as a powerful anti-inflammatory herb 2000 years ago in the Holy Bible (see our Seminar 'Health from the Bible').

IN A NUTSHELL

If you are one of those more than 10% of the U.S. population hit by eczema, trust nature's kingdom of powerful remedies and modalities to relieve itching, dryness, swelling and infection of the skin. As indicated in this scientifically verified elaboration.

19. SUFFERING FROM PHOBIA? WHICH PHOBIA?

THE PHILOSOPHY BEHIND

More than 3 quarters of all health issues in our industrialized world are ´chronically´ unsolved. One of the reasons is that most of us only focus on physical symptoms of respective health issues. Overlooking the fact that any living species on this planet – man being no exception – is an *ecologic* phenomenon. I.e. each health issue needs to be considered also from a mental point of view, in relation to its physical status.

With special reference to the fact that there are many mental criteria involved in our ecologic existence most of us are not necessarily familiar with.

One of these mental disorders are *phobias*, i.e. a type of anxiety disorder with intense and exaggerated fears about a certain situation, place, a living creature or an object. Dependent on a particular trigger, these phobias may sometimes lead even to panic attacks.

Related to following potential *physical* effects, to round up the ecologic phenomenon.

Inter alia,
- headache
- sweating
- dry mouth
- confusion/disorientation
- dizziness
- chest pains/tightness
- accelerated heartbeat
- nausea
- hot flushes/chills
- abnormal breathing
- choking sensation
- trembling

Not only this. According to the *World Mental Health Survey* by the World Health Organization (WHO), more than 60% of those having a phobia during lifetime, usually also have another mental health problem such as, inter alia,
- depression

- bipolar disorder
- another type of anxiety disorder
- impulse control disorder
- substance use disorder

Thereby, phobias can be the result of traumatic events.

In the U.S. alone, there are almost 20 million citizens suffering from phobias, according to the *Anxiety and Depression Association of America (ADDA)*. With up to almost 10% of U.S. citizens being hit by any type of phobia per year.

Internationally, based on research at, inter alia, the *University Medical Center* at the *Georg-August University* in Göttingen, Germany, some 10% of the general population not only were struck by a specific phobia within last 12 months but had a specific phobia during lifetime.

To be developed mostly already in younger years (i.e. in early childhood - about 8 years of age), teenage years and early adulthood, but rarely after the age of 30. Although most phobias come and go during childhood/adolescence, some may well be found even in adulthood.

Thereby, children may express their fear by, inter alia,
- refusing to speak/move
- clinging physically to parent/object
- having tantrums
- crying

Interestingly, based on the above mentioned *World Mental Health Survey*, females are more affected than males.

TYPES OF PHOBIAS – SCIENTIFICALLY VERIFIED

Basically, ADDA differs between different types of phobias according to. certain fears as anxiety disorders. With *acrophobia* (fear of heights) and zoophobia (fear of animals) as the most common specific phobias.

Verified by international research at, inter alia,
- *University of Queensland* in Brisbane, Australia
- *University of Quebec Outaouais* in Gatineau, Canada
- *Ruhr University Bochum* in Bochum, Germany
- *Johns Hopkins Bloomberg School of Public Health* & *Johns Hopkins School of Medicine* in Baltimore, MD
- *University of Pennsylvania* in Philadelphia, PA
- *University of California* in Los Angeles, CA

- *Stockholm University* and *Karolinska Institute,* both in Stockholm, Sweden
- *University of Groningen* in Groningen, The Netherlands
- *University of Otago* in Dunedin, New Zealand
- *Federation University* in Ballarat, Australia
- *Al-Qadisiya University* in Al Diwaniya, Iraq
- *University of Sao Paulo* in Sao Paulo, Brazil
- *Ulster University* in Londonderry, UK
- *Katholieke Universiteit Leuven* in Leuven, Belgium
- *University Medical Center* in Göttingen, Germany
- *University of Ibadan* in Ibadan, Nigeria
- *Peking University* in Beijing, China
- *Balamand University* in Beirut, Lebanon
- *Wroclaw Medical University* in Wroclaw, Poland
- *Monash University* in Melbourne, Australia
- *Universidad Cayetano Hereidia* in St. Martin de Porres, Peru
- *El Bosque University & CES University* - both in Bogota, Colombia
- *Universidade Nova de Lisboa* in Lisboa, Portugal

As a variety, let´s focus now on a sample of different phobia types, as follows (in alphabetical order).

Acrophobia

This type of phobia is an extreme fear of heights and one of the most common types which may happen to 5% of the population.

With the effect that those concerned usually are shy to step on a ladder, bridge or balcony, or enter a plane.

Physical symptoms in such cases are, inter alia,
- heart palpitations
- sweating
- shortness of breath
- nausea

Aquaphobia

This kind refers to an extreme/irrational fear of any types of water like high tides, rapids or murky lakes. (Usually not, however, ´harmless´ bodies of water like bathtubs or pools.)

Physical symptoms in such a case are, inter alia,
- rapid heartbeat

- trembling/shaking
- sweating
- shallow breathing
- dry mouth
- butterflies in stomach
- chills
- dizziness
- confusion/disorientation
- nausea

Arachnophobia

As one of the most usual types of phobias, it is an intense/paralyzing fear of arachnids like spiders and others. In many cases developed already in childhood. Triggered even in cases where these arachnids are seen just on a picture instead of reality.

With physical symptoms such as, inter alia,
- increased heart rate
- shaking
- breathing difficulty
- dizziness
- fainting
- sweating
- nausea

Emetophobia

This type of anxiety disorder is the fear of vomiting. As such it may give those affected the feeling of being sick themselves or others may get sick with vomiting.

It can develop after a traumatic experience with vomiting involved.

In many cases, emetophobia is connected with *depression*.

Also, it may be connected with other mental health issues like generalized anxiety or obsessive-compulsive disorder.

As far as physical symptoms are concerned, these are basically
- nausea
- vomiting
  and
- weight loss (as a result)

Thalassophobia

In this case, the affected person may be anxious about the emptiness or vastness of the ocean (or other *deep* bodies of water) or living species in it – sometimes of both.

This can happen in different situations like
- visiting beaches
- walking in the shallow waters of the ocean
- riding on boats
  or just
- in proximity of an ocean

This may be prevalent already in early years e.g. when learning to swim or even from news coverages about, inter alia, shark attacks or tsunami.

Related to physical symptoms such as, inter alia,
- elevated heart rate
- sweating
- faster breathing

However, it can also lead to panic attack with additional physical symptoms, such as, inter alia,
- heart palpitations
- rapid breathing/hyperventilation
- feeling of choking
- trembling/shaking
- nausea with/without vomiting

Potentially related to the feeling of fainting and even the feeling to die.

Finally,

Zoophobia

as an umbrella term for the intense fear of certain animals, causing manifold stress and reduction of life quality. Which affects some people with fear/anxiety when seeing or thinking about animals.

Besides *arachnophobia* which we covered already above, this umbrella term *zoophobia* also incorporates, inter alia (again in alphabetical order):

- *apiphobia* (fear of bees)
- *cynophobia* (fear of dogs)
- *entomophobia* (fear of insects)

- *ichthyophobia* (fear of fish)
- *murophobia* (fear of rats and mice)
- *ornithophobia* (fear of birds)
- *ophidiophobia* (fear of snakes)

With following potential physical symptoms involved:
- increased heart rate
- dizziness
- shallow/fast breathing
- numbness
- confusion
- chills
- dry mouth
- trembling/shaking
- sweating
- nausea

Children affected by zoophobia usually are known for expressing their anxiety with, inter alia,
- screaming
- crying
- becoming still/silent
- attempting to hide between persons or objects
- having tantrum

NATURAL SELF-MANAGEMENT OF PHOBIAS

Best way is certainly to dodge the source of fear behind the phobia to stay in control. However, if you can't avoid, try following modalities to cope with the situation. Inter alia...

- Mindfulness

Stay in present moment the trigger hits to reduce tension by notice and focus on physical sensations, breathing, or surroundings.

- Self-compassion

Being self-compassionate may well reduce stress related to the anxiety.

- Breathing exercises

If you are breathing slowly and steadily, this may stop hyperventilation to return to calmness. Especially, when anxiety is intensifying.

- Distraction

Try to distract yourself by focusing on different situations by, e.g., reading a book, listening to music or talk to a dear person like a family member or friend.

IN A NUTSHELL

Phobias – one of the most common mental health disorders – are affecting more than 260 million people worldwide. Some 20 million in the U.S. alone. Fortunately, there are natural ways of self-management, as you learn in this chapter.

20. WHICH NUTRITION TO STAY IN SHAPE?

THE PHILOSOPHY BEHIND

As we know, our health and longevity is resting on 2 basic pillars: physical exercise and healthy nutrition. Leaves us with the question which nutritious food to reach this goal. Especially, as most non-age-related deaths and diseases are the result of 'chronic', i.e. unsolved health problems. With heart failure on top of the list, followed by cancer and diabetes.

HEALTHY DIET – SCIENTIFICALLY VALIDATED

To avoid and get out of this vicious cycle, respectively, we may follow the USDA food pattern as recommended by the U.S. National Institute on Aging. While we cannot cover the whole spectrum of nutrition in this brief chapter, let's focus at least on following sample of some basic nutrients.

Whole grains

Refined grain being milled as flour or meal is missing bran and germ, also stripped of equally vital B-vitamins, fiber and iron. On the other hand, whole grain contains these nutrients vital for different body functions such as, inter alia, regulating our immune system, to carry oxygen in the blood just as balancing blood sugar.

That's why, inter alia, the *American Heart Association* recommends whole grain with high priority. Especially, as heart failure is the no. 1 in our statistics of premature death.

Fiber

Equally important, according to the *American Heart Association* is to consume enough dietary fiber. To manage blood cholesterol and cut down the risk of heart disease – as well as of type 2 diabetes and obesity.

Doing justice accordingly, whole grain just as vegetables, as well as beans and pulses may be on your weekly menu.

Beans & pulses

Beans and pulses not only contain fiber, but are also a vital source of vitamins and minerals as well as vital protein.

As scientifically verified at, inter alia, *Purdue University* in West Lafayette, IN, and *Bastyr University* in Kenmore, WA.

Protein

Based on research at, inter alia, the

- *University of Minnesota* in Minneapolis, MN
- *Technische Universität Dresden* in Dresden, Germany
- *University of Birmingham* in Birmingham, UK
- *University of Exeter Medical School* in Exeter, UK
- *Emory University* in Atlanta, GA

protein may not only balance blood sugar for better diabetes management but also for weight management, and is beneficial for our cardiovascular health.

Green leafy vegetables

According to the *U.S. Department of Agriculture (USDA)* dark green leafy vegetables are an excellent source of nutrition, based on its content of vitamins, minerals and antioxidants.

With special reference to its inherent vitamin K for prevention of osteoporosis and folate to fight cancer.

Same source of recommendation (USDA) also promotes...

Plant foods

... in general as it is not only helpful for weight loss but also in terms of health in general, by cutting down the risk of debilitating health issues such as diabetes and cardiovascular disease.

Unsaturated fats

... as to be found in, inter alia, in avocados, vegetable oils and...

Oily fish

... are equally important. Scientifically verified by, inter alia, the

- *University of Arizona* in Tucson, AZ

- *University of South Dakota* in Sioux Falls, SD
- *Pennsylvania State University in University Park, PA*
- *University of Southampton* in Southampton, UK,
- *Sapienza University* in Rome, Italy
- *University of Modena and Reggio Emilia* in Modena, Italy)

Additionally validated by the *U.S. Department of Agriculture.*

With special reference to its inherent omega-3 fatty acids which may not only reduce risk of cardiovascular disease but also manage early stages of Alzheimer's and Parkinson's disease.

Extra virgin olive oil

Based on international research at, inter alia,

- *Harvard TH Chan School of Public Health* in Boston, MA
- *University of Jaen* in Jaen, Spain
- *University of Padova* in Padova, Italy
- *University of Seville* in Sevilla, Spain
- *University of Zaragoza* in Zaragoza, Spain
- *Universidad de la Republica* in Montevideo, Uruguay
- *University of Granada School of Medicine* in Granada, Spain
- *University of Crete* in Heraklion, Greece
- *University of Navarra* in Pamplona, Spain
- *University of Freiburg* in Freiburg, Germany
- *University of Bristol* in Bristol, UK

this Mediterranean 'wonder food' is helpful for our heart, blood pressure and weight management, etc., when added to our diet such as vegetables and salads.

Water

To drink enough water is not only an asset for weight management. But also to cut down the risk of kidney stones, body overheat, constipation, mood change, etc.

According to the U.S. *Centers for Disease Control and Prevention (CDC).*

Even more important – especially for elder people - to avoid dehydration as a risk factor for health issues in general. Based on research at, inter alia,

- *University of California* in Los Angeles, CA

- *Radboud University Nijmegen Medical Center* in Nijmegen, Netherlands
- *Vanderbilt University School of Medicine* in Nashville, TN
- *University of California* in San Francisco, CA
- *Birzeit University* in Birzeit, Palestine
- *University of Iowa* in Iowa City, IA
- *Edinburgh Napier University* in Edinburgh, UK
- *Purdue University* in West Lafayette, IN
- *Bangor University* in Bangor, UK
- *St. Luke's International University* in Tokyo, Japan
- *Brigham Young University* in Provo, UT
- *University of East Anglia* in Norwich, UK
- *University of Liverpool* in Liverpool, UK

Coffee

Moderate consumption of 3-5 cups a day by adults in general (2 cups in cases of pregnancy and lactating) may cut the risk of

- diabetes type 2
- cardiovascular disease
- Alzheimer's disease
- Parkinson's disease

According to research at, inter alia, *Gazi University* in Turkey's capital Ankara.

Herbs & Spices

To round up your healthy nutrition, you may also consider following herbs and spices.

- Curcumin

as part of the historically/biblically belauded herb *turmeric* is not only known for its anti-inflammatory property but for our health in general.

Based on research at, inter alia, the *Universidad de Granada* in Granada, Spain.

Just as

- Garlic

which is anti-inflammatory as well, along with many other antioxidant and antimicrobial benefits.

According to research at, inter alia, *Shanghai Jiao Tong University* in Shanghai and *Yat-sen University* in Guangzhou - both China – as well as *Stellenbosch University* in Cape Town, South Africa.

- Ginger

with its anti-inflammatory power especially during our aging process, along with preventing oxidative stress.

Based on research at, inter alia, *Universiti Kebangsaan Malaysia Medical Centre* in Kuala Lumpur, Malaysia.

Leaves us finally with the question,

WHICH KIND OF FOOD TO LIMIT/AVOID

- Processed food

Ultra-processed food may increase the risk of many different and debilitating diseases such as, inter alia, cancer, depression and irritable bowel syndrome.

According to research at, inter alia, *Deakin University* in Geelong, Australia, and *Bjorknes University College* in Norway's capital Oslo.

This comes even worse with red and processed meat, raising the mortality rate.

Based on research at, inter alia,
- *Harvard T.H. Chan School of Public Health & Harvard Medical School* in Boston, MA
- *Fudan University in Shanghai & Huazhong University of Science and Technology* in Wuhan – both China
- *Ohio University* in Athens, OH
- *Universidad Autonoma de Madrid* in Spain's capital Madrid

- Sugar

Dietary sugar, high fructose corn syrup and dextrose may well harm our cardiovascular system.

According to research at, inter alia, the *University of California* in Davis, CA.

Even worse:

- Sugary drinks

which, according to the U.S. *Centers for Disease Control and Prevention (CDC)* may elicit, inter alia,
- heart disease
- diabetes type 2
- kidney disease
- weight gain/obesity
- non-alcoholic liver disease
- gout
- tooth decay

IN A NUTSHELL

Besides physical exercise, healthy diet is one of the 2 pillars our health and longevity rests on. Doing justice accordingly, the U.S. National Institute of Aging recommends a food pattern developed by the U.S. Department of Agriculture. Including, inter alia, a variety of fruits and vegetables, whole grains, unsaturated fats, seafood, etc. With special reference to healthy Mediterranean style eating. All scientifically validated.

21. BENEFITS OF CARDIO FOR YOUR HEALTH

THE PHILOSOPHY BEHIND

As you may know already very well, to stay/become healthy for long life, 2 basic parameters are inevitable: healthy diet and physical exercise. When focusing on latter,

Cardiovascular exercise

(also going by the brief medical term *cardio*) plays a major role especially for our heart, by improving our heart rate.

Not only.

In fact, according to, inter alia, *Victoria University* in Melbourne, Australia, cardiovascular exercise has not only a very comprehensive benefit for strengthening our heart for bumping faster but for our health in general. Including, inter alia,

- boosting immune system
- improving sleep patterns
- lowering cholesterol
- increasing bone density
- preventing/managing high blood pressure
- lowering stress
- preventing/managing diabetes
- managing weight by burning fat and calories
- increasing stamina
- increasing breathing rate

While these *physical* benefits may well prevail, we don't want to overlook also the *mental* benefits of cardio.

Such as a brisk walk of only 30 minutes has a positive impact on depression and anxiety.

TYPES OF CARDIO – SCIENTIFICALLY VALIDATED

According to research at, inter alia, *Harvard Medical School* in Boston, MA, *VU University Medical Center* in Amsterdam, The Netherlands, and *Durban University of Technology* in Durban, South Africa,

- *running*
- *walking*
- *cycling*
- *swimming*

are excellent forms of cardiovascular ('cardio') exercise , as the heart (and lungs) are working harder in these cases.

Scientifically verified by the U.S. Centers for Disease Control and Prevention.

Thereby, at least 75 minutes of vigorous intensity or 150 minutes of moderate intensity exercise per week are to prefer. Verified by research also at *Harvard Medical School* in Cambridge, MA.

According to research at the *Norwegian University of Science and Technology* in Trondheim, Norway, higher fitness levels can cut down the risk of coronary artery disease by 50% for otherwise healthy people, without a history of cardiovascular disease.

To be rounded off by walking 30 minutes a day or 60 minutes every other day – for health in general and heart support specifically. According to the *Preventive Medicine Research Institute* in Sausalito, California.

Aerobic physical exercise can prevent arterial stiffening to avoid cardiovascular events, as scientifically verified at the *University College London,* UK.

We may also not want to overlook the relationship between muscle mass and cardiovascular health in general.

Because according to research at the *University of Canberra* in Canberra, Australia, the *University of Athens* in Athens, Greece, and the *Centro de Investigacion Biomedica en Red de Salud Mental* in Spain's capital Madrid, cardiovascular health has to be seen in relationship to muscle mass. Especially in cases of males aged 45 and over. With reference to the fact that starting at age 30, muscle mass tends to decrease by 3-5% every 10 years.

I.e. if males are losing muscle mass, their risk of cardiovascular disease and related premature death is rising. Although the researchers didn't find the cause behind, the results of their study needs to be taken serious. However, the benefit of physical exercise is not one-sided in terms of gender.

According to research at the *University of Southern Denmark* in Odense, Denmark, untrained females with high blood pressure benefitted from playing football (soccer) not only in terms of bone density and body fat percentage but also blood pressure.

Based on research at the *University of Paris* in France's capital, we have to differ between sports based physical activity strengthening the neuro baroreflex avoiding cardiovascular issues, and strenuous exertion on the job.

The latter with a negative effect – on arterial stiffness (mechanical baroreflex) and the neural baroreflex, leading to heart rhythm issues. This does not mean that any physical movement at work is negative for our heart; rather, chronic strenuous activity (like heavy load lifting) could well be.

This kind of exercise is especially important for heart failure patients to cut down their risk of hospitalization and death with exercise intensity. E.g., on stationary bicycle or walking on treadmill for 25-30 minutes many days during the week. According to research at *Henry Ford Hospital* in Detroit, Michigan.

IN A NUTSHELL

Cardiovascular exercise (also going by the brief medical term *cardio*) is not only vital to support a healthy heart but comprehensively to stay/become healthy for long life in general. As you learn in this chapter, scientifically validated.

22. DIABETES: TREAT BLOOD SUGAR WITH NATURE

THE PHILOSOPHY BEHIND

The U.S. is worldwide # 1 in conventional medicine. Spending most for medicine in the industrialized world, with $3.5 trillion per year, according to the *Centers for Disease Control and Prevention (CDC)*.

Despite of that, more than 80% of non-age-related deaths are the consequence of unsolved health problems (according to the *World Health Organization – WHO*). With diabetes 2 in top region, along with heart failure and cancer.

In fact, according to the *Centers for Disease Control and Prevention (CDC)*, 30 million U.S. adults, i.e. some 12% of our population in total are diagnosed with diabetes 2. Another 84 million U.S. adults are prediabetic, i.e. with higher-than-normal blood sugar levels.

Unfortunately, there is no synthetic drug on the market to stop this debilitating health issue. Rather, the most prescribed synthetic drug with 120 million prescriptions worldwide, comes with a minimum of 69 side effects, according to its producer (pharma giant *Bristol Myers Squibb*) but no cure.

LOWER BLOOD SUGAR – SCIENTIFICALLY VALIDATED

The only chance lies with lowering the blood sugar level.

Not only for appropriate diabetes management but also to avoid debilitating consequences of high blood sugar. Such as, inter alia,

- impairment of vision and even blindness
- heart attack/stroke
- kidney failure
- damage to nervous system

If tried again with synthetics, new side effects and health issues may be the result. A vicious cycle.

Other than adjusting your nutrition and other lifestyle factors the natural way to lower high blood sugar level. As follows.

Nutrition

- Quantity & quality of carbohydrates

According to research at, inter alia, the *University of Minnesota* in Minneapolis, MN, eat low-carbohydrate & high-protein food to cut your blood sugar level.

With special reference to complex carbohydrates such as whole grain oats and sweet potatoes.

In this context, also

- Soluble fiber

is important, as it slows down the breakdown of carbohydrates and the pace of the absorption of related sugar.

This kind of fiber we find, inter alia, in
- whole grains (like brown rice, etc.)
- fruits
- vegetables

- Low glycemic index foods

To take a look at the glycemic index of the food you consume is important, since the glycemic index is measuring foods in terms of rising blood sugar levels. Therefore, it is relevant to swallow foods with an index below of 55. Such as, inter alia,
- non-starchy vegetables
- legumes
- nuts & seeds
- leafy greens
- quinoa
- sweet potatoes
- low-fat milk
- fish
- etc.

According to research, inter alia, in Bucharest, Romania, at
- *N. Paulescu National Institute of Diabetes, Nutrition and Metabolic Diseases,*
- *Carol Davila University of Medicine,* and the
- *Foundation for Healthy Nutrition*

- Water

Staying hydrated is not only important for our health in general but to cut down blood sugar in particular, as it supports kidneys getting rid of extra sugar in the urine.

Avoiding fruit juices and other sugary drinks (including soda and fruit juices) at the same time.

Based on research at, inter alia, the *Worcestershire Royal Hospital* in Worcester, UK.

Although not directly part of our nutrition,

- Herbs

such as, inter alia,
  - green tea
  - cinnamon
  - bitter melon
  - fenugreek
  - American ginseng
  - aloe vera

do have some relevance in this nutritional context to boost diet with essential nutrients with respect to controlling levels of blood sugar.

Other lifestyle factors

- Stress management

Unlike manifold assumptions, stress does have a severe impact on blood sugar, as stress hormones released by the body under tension may well raise the level of blood sugar.

Based on research at, inter alia, *Kangwon National University* in Chuncheon, South Korea.

- Weight control

Being overweight supports diabetes in a negative sense. To avoid, regular consumption of fruits and vegetables, as well as exercise is helpful.

According to research at *George Washington University* in Rockville, MD, already 7% of weight loss can lower the risk of diabetes by 58%.

- Exercise

Thereby, exercise is not only good for weight control but also increases insulin sensitivity.

According to research at, inter alia, *Cardiff University* in Cardiff, UK.

This implies the importance also of sound

- Sleep

as a lack of sleep could raise blood sugar level with respect to insulin resistance. Especially in early morning.

IN A NUTSHELL

Diabetes 2 is one of the top non-age-related diseases and deaths in the U.S. with more than 30 million adults diagnosed, plus more than 80 million prediabetics. Unfortunately, with no synthetic solution. Therefore, we tend to nature's answers of cutting down blood sugar.

23. HOW RELIEVE CHRONIC PAIN NATURALLY?

THE PHILOSOPHY BEHIND

Derived from the Greek word *ponos* (meaning 'body fights back') the term *pain* has been coined by the ancient Greek physician and philosopher *Hippocrates* 400 B.C. as the neurological signal that 'something is wrong in this/that part of the body'.

According to the *World Health Organization (WHO),* scientifically verified, inter alia, by the *Harvard School of Public Health* in Cambridge, MA, pain is related to certain diseases and the most debilitating disability of mankind today.

Affecting some 20% of the adult population in the U.S, according to the U.S. *Centers for Disease Control and Prevention (CDC).*

According to research at, inter alia, *National University of Singapore* & *Nanyang Technological University* – both located in Singapore, China – we understand that the term *chronic* refers to pain lasting longer than 3 months.

Not only this, chronic pain, due to its complexity, comes along with additional health conditions, physically and mentally. Such as, inter alia, sleep problems, depression, and even social isolation.

With the result that synthetics (painkiller drugs) are representing the 4th leading premature death rate, according to the *U.S. Institutes of Health* – without solving the underlying problem.

U.S. NAVY'S NEW MISSION "ALTERNATIVE MEDICINE"

That's one reason why the U.S. Navy has launched a new mission called 'Alternative Medicine', after the military and especially the veterans could not solve their *Post-Traumatic Stress Disorder (PTSD)* with conventional medicine.

Commented by highly decorated Army Col. Richard Petri in his capacity of chief of physical medicine and integrative health services at the *William Beaumont Army Medical Center* in Fort Bliss, Texas: "If we don't change our practices, health care in the military will bankrupt the military."

NATURAL TECHNIQUES – SCIENTIFICALLY VALIDATED

Doing justice accordingly, we will not cover natural remedies for replacement of synthetic painkiller drugs in this brief elaboration, but we shall focus strictly on natural techniques, with special reference to self-management by the patient. In order to reduce and control the chronic pain.

One of these techniques may be

- **Massage**

Based on research at, inter alia, the *University of California* in Los Angeles (UCLA), this form of soft-tissue manipulation may lower back pain.

Additionally, massage may help with

- improvement of circulation
- reducing inflammation
- relaxation
- improving posture

- **Acupuncture**

Similar, according to the U.S. *National Center for Complementary and Integrative Health,* this type of natural therapy may not only help to relieve pain in the lower back as well, but also with

- pain relief in general
- reducing inflammation
- reducing muscle spasm
- relaxation

More directly for

- **Relaxation**

there are techniques to relieve muscle spasms and tensions and even more, they can release *endorphins,* our body's – yes – natural painkillers.

According to, inter alia, the *West Suffolk NHS Foundation Trust* in Suffolk, UK.

Which techniques for relaxation?

Inter alia,

-   Progressive muscle relaxation
    to relax each group of muscles for 10 seconds, head to toe.

-   Deep breathing
    to relieve tension by relaxed breathing techniques also named 'box breathing' which means deep breathing in order to turn back breathing in stressful situations to normal. Especially when the body is in a 'fight-or-flight' mode.

-   Calming
    to dedicate certain times for relaxation for, e.g., reading a book, crafting or simply taking a warm bath. And simply spending a couple of minutes to think about calming situations like, e.g., a sunny day in nature.

-   ***Mind-body connection***

E.g.,

-   Yoga

This ancient Indian technique can well support you to release tension, experiencing calmness and clarity, and to relax.

Even more, according to research at *McGill University* in Montreal, Canada, this ancient and safe technique may also relieve the pain.

-   Tai chi

As another form of Indian-Ayurvedic culture, in combination with relaxation and breathing techniques, also improves mood based on the concentration required for this technique

Based on research at, inter alia, the
-   *University of Technology Sydney* in Sydney, Australia
-   *University of Duisburg-Essen* in Essen, Germany
    and
-   *Shanghai University of Traditional Chinese Medicine* in Shanghai, China

this technique may well relieve chronic pain, with special reference to lower back pain, rheumatic arthritis and osteoporosis.

IN A NUTSHELL

Chronic pain is one of the most debilitating health issues in our industrialized society. In most cases treated synthetically with painkiller drugs. Along with side effects, physically and mentally, but no cure. In this blog you learn about techniques to relieve and control chronic pain naturally.

24. WHICH EXERCISES FOR YOUR HEALTH?

THE PHILOSOPHY BEHIND

As you may have learned from our previous publications and other presentations, to support our health and longevity, physical exercise plays a decisive role, besides healthy diet. Especially, as exercise basically strengthens different groups of muscles in our body and, along with cardiovascular exercise, supports our heart, cardiovascular system in particular.

In this blog we shall focus on physical exercises you can follow easily even at your home. With moderate intensity 30 minutes per day 5 times a week, or 3 times a week vigorously. Repeatedly.

TYPES OF EXERCISE – VERIFIED BY RESEARCH

Based on scientific research at the *American College of Sports Medicine (ACSM)* and supported by the *American Council on Exercise,* different types of exercise are recommended. Cutting out 'profane' types of these exercises (like running and swimming, etc.), we shall cover half a dozen of more 'exotic' ones in following.

Let's start with...

Body Weight Squats

To support the strength of lower body and core, with its effect on hips, buttocks, abs, calves, shins, and thighs.

To do:

- Have your feet standing little bit wider apart, with toes showing outward.
- Support your back by having abdominal muscles engaged.
- Keep a flat back by bending the knees as if taking a seat, shifting the hips back.
- Lower down to the bottom until thighs are parallel to the floor.
- Pushing feet through in order to straighten your back up to position you started.
- Keep shoulders back, with hands down and palms facing in.
- Inhale into squat and exhale when you stand up again.

Glute bridge/stability

This type supports the muscles in your back – the posterior chain.

To do:

- Lie on back with knees bent, having feet flat on floor.
- Contract abdominal muscles and buttocks in order to raise hips above floor.
- Go back to starting position.

Side planks

This type of exercise supports building core strength for lowering back pain. With its effect on hips, abdominal muscles and buttocks.

To do:

- Lie down on your right side with outstretched legs, and with elbow under right shoulder.
- Engaging the abdominal muscles, lift hips and knees above bottom, head and body being aligned.
- Do this for 15-20 seconds, without dropping head, shoulders or hips.
- Return to bottom slowly, switching to the left, repeating again.

Knee tucks

With using an exercise ball, do it this way:

- With stomach on the exercise/stability ball, hands and feet on floor.
- Crawl forward on hands getting knees to rest on the ball, feet lifted above ground. With hands resting underneath shoulders.
- Rolling knees forward and curl into chest.
- Pushing knees back slowly in order to get back to starting position.

Pike roll-out

This is another exercise type you may carry out with a stability ball. To challenge your arm, shoulder, and abdominal muscles.

To do:

- Lie down on the ball, hands and feet on bottom.

- Roll with the ball forward, with flexed toes resting on it. Thereby, keep straight, arms straight under shoulders, and with palms on bottom flat.
- Hips in line with shoulders, straight head and back between arms.
- Hinging at hips, buttocks lifted towards ceiling, have legs straight with toes flexed on ball.
- Slow back down to position as you started.

Lunges

This is again in favor of buttocks, hips, and abdominal muscles.

To do:

- Standing upright, having feet together.
- Bending the knee of the supportive leg down to floor.
- Stepping one leg forward into long stride, bend knee, place foot on bottom flat.
- Using muscles of forward leg, pushing back to standing.
- Then do same with second leg.

IN A NUTSHELL

Our health and longevity basically rests on 2 pillars: healthy diet and physical activity. In this blog, we focus on half a dozen of physical exercises recommended by the *American College of Sports Medicine (ACSM)* and the *American Council on Exercise*. With special reference to health of our heart and cardiovascular system, respectively - #1 of non-age-related premature death in our modern society.

25. FIGHT FLU & COLD WITH NATURE

THE PHILOSOPHY BEHIND

The Covid-19 pandemic tended to let us overlook the fact that this viral infection has got a close relative we know since long: the ordinary flu (influenza) as a respiratory health issue as well.

Especially, as this close relationship comes in both cases with more or less same symptoms. Such as
- Shortness of breath
- Fever
- Sore throat
- Headache
- Fatigue
- Muscle pain/body aches
- Running/stuffy nose

To be added, as far as corona is concerned, in terms of
- New loss of taste or smell
- Nausea/vomiting
- Diarrhea

NATURAL FLU REMEDIES – SCIENTIFICALLY VALIDATED

These symptomatic similarities may not let us forget that our ancestors have known already natural remedies against viral infections for thousands of years and which, to be sure, have been scientifically verified manifold today.

Just to focus on a small sample of these remedies from nature's kingdom of health:

Echinacea

There are anti-viral compounds in the roots of this herb to support the immune response. Even for newborns younger than 2 weeks old.

Based on research at, inter alia, the *University of Basrah* in Basrah, Iraq.

Another powerful herbal root offering the same effect for our health is the one herb native to America and Asia

Ginseng

according to research at, inter alia, *St. John's University* in Queens, NY.

Licorice

root is also an important anti-viral and immune-mediating herb to fight viral respiratory infections.

Based on research at, inter alia, *Beijing University of Chinese Medicine* in China's capital Beijing.

Not to overlook another powerful root to fight viral infections –

Star anise

with its anti-viral compounds, including spirooligananone A & B, and shikimic acid.

According to research at, inter alia, *Bengasi School of Technology* in Hugli, and *Gupta College of Technological Sciences* in Asansol – both India.

Aqueous

Dandelion

may also reduce viral infection of the lungs.

Based on research at, inter alia, the *University of the Chinese Academy of Sciences* in China's capital Beijing.

Milkwort

species *polygala karensium* is also fighting flu viruses with its antiviral compound *xanthones*.

According to research at, inter alia, *Chosun University* in Gwangju, South Korea.

Similar the effect of

Cinnamon

bark as used with its antiviral effect in traditional Japanese herbal medicine named *maoto*.

Based on research at, inter alia, *Fukuoka University Hospital* in Fukuoka, Japan.

Elderberries

This fruit (like some other berries) is powerful to tackle the flu, as it contains immune-modulating polyphenols.

According to research at, inter alia, *St. John's University College of Pharmacy & Health Sciences* in Queens, NY.

IN A NUTSHELL

The viral infection of COVID-19 is not a unique health issue but a relative of our well known virally infectious flu (influenza). Tackled by our ancestors for thousands of years with natural remedies, manifold scientifically verified today. As covered in this chapter with a small sample from nature's kingdom.

26. AVOID DIABETIC DEATH WITH COFFEE & TEA?

THE PHILOSOPHY BEHIND

According to the *World Health Organization (WHO)*, 86% of non-age-related premature deaths in the industrialized countries are the consequence of 'chronic' (unsolved) health problems. In the U.S. alone, more than 60% of U.S. adults are affected with at least one, and 40% with 2 or more chronic diseases, according to estimates of the U.S. *Centers for Disease Control and Prevention (CDC)*.

With diabetes 2 being in the upper range of the statistics. Based on the fact that, according to *CDC* statistics, 10% of U.S. adults are suffering from this debilitating disease. In many cases as the cause behind of other debilitating health issues such as, inter alia, cancer, circulatory diseases, dementia and bone fractures.

Unfortunately yet, conventional medicine hasn't found a solution for this vicious cycle yet. With special reference to the fact that world's most prescribed diabetic drug - according to its producer - not only comes with more than 80 side effects but above all, with no cure. Reinforcing the vicious cycle.

This, however, doesn't mean that nature doesn't offer us any solutions for this 'chronic' disease at all. Since our globe, the Earth, is a perfect ecologic system, strictly based on natural laws, there may well be natural answers on our planet to escape this fate of vicious cycle.

NUTRITIONAL ADJUSTMENTS – SCIENTIFICALLY VERIFIED

Besides factors such physical activity, sound sleep, high blood pressure management and non-smoking, etc., healthy diet has become increasingly an issue to manage diabetes naturally.

With special reference to our daily nutrition according to, inter alia, following recent international scientific findings.

Green Tea

E.g., research at *Kyushu University* in Fukuoka, Japan, suggests that green tea may well reduce the risk of developing diabetes at all.

Improving insulin sensitivity and glucose control, as verified also by the *Third Military Medical University* in Chongqing, People's Republic of China.

Similar the situation with

Coffee

which may lower the risk of diabetes as well, as verified at, inter alia, *Southampton University & Southampton General Hospital* in Southampton, UK, and the *University of Edinburgh* in Edinburgh, UK.

More than that, according to the U.S. *National Institutes of Health,* coffee consumption may even reduce the risk of related mortality.

Leaves us with the question: how much green tea and/or coffee to consume to avoid premature death from diabetes?

To reduce the risk by...

- 51% - drink 2-3 cups of green tea & at least 2 cups of coffee per day
- 58% - drink 4+ cups of green tea & 1 cup of coffee per day
- 63% - drink 4+ cups of green tea & at least 2 cups of coffee per day

With drinking only 2+ cups of coffee per day, risk of premature mortality may decrease at least by more than 40%.

According to scientific findings at *Kyushu University* in Fukuoka and *Hakujyuji Hospital* in Kamisu, both Japan.

IN A NUTSHELL

Diabetes is one of the leading 'chronic' diseases responsible for premature (non-age-related) deaths in our industrialized society. While conventional medicine could not solve this problem yet, recent international scientific evidence suggests that nature may give us some answers with tea and coffee.

27. WALK AWAY FROM DIABETES

THE PHILOSOPHY BEHIND

According to latest statistics of the World Health Organization (WHO), 86% of non-age-related premature death (with 2 million only in the U.S.) & 77% of all ailments in general in the industrialized world are the consequence of unsolved (chronic) disease. With diabetes being third behind heart failure and cancer.

Based inter alia on the fact that the most prescribed medication for diabetes worldwide – according to its pharmaceutical producer – comes with more than 80 side effects, but no cure.

NATURAL WAY OUT – SCIENTIFICALLY VERIFIED

While the American Diabetes Association recommended already 150 minutes of moderate exercise per week to ward off diabetes, now we learn from a scientific meta-analysis of 7 studies carried out by the *Old Dominion University* in Norfolk, VA, with special reference to blood sugar that

-   2-5 minutes of light walking 60-90 minutes after a meal

can well cut down the risk of developing diabetes 2.

Scientifically verified also by the *University of Limerick* in Limerick, Ireland.

Besides the fact that even standing after a meal instead of sitting is already in favor of reducing the risk.

By smoothing blood sugar spikes after the meal.

Should you not be in the position to manage that, e.g. when involved in office work, then you should e.g. walk up and down the staircase of the office building several times after lunch or have a phone meeting, while walking around the block, etcetera,

IN A NUTSHELL

Diabetes 2, indicated in top regions of World Health Organization's global statistics of unsolved/chronic disease, has not found any effective solution with medication yet. While international medical science has come up with a challenging and striking lifestyle factor, we may not want to overlook it.

28. HOW TREAT MS NATURALLY?

THE PHILOSOPHY BEHIND

- Multiple Sclerosis (MS) is the attack of the immune system on our central nervous system (CNS) which is made up of our brain, spinal cord and optic nerves.
- Accordingly, this attack is disrupting flow of information in the brain & its transmission between brain and body.
- While, according to the U.S. *National Multiple Sclerosis Society,* the cause behind is not yet scientifically verified, certain factors like genetics, infections, immunology and epidemiology may play a role.
- Affecting some 1 million citizens in the U.S.
- Thereby, MS causes inflammation in the body, along with physical and mental symptoms such as, inter alia,
    - fatigue
    - pain
    - reduced mobility
    - numbness/tingling of arms/legs
    - itching
    - sexual problems
    - dizziness
    - cognitive problems
    - urinary tract infection
    - osteoporosis
    - depression
- Conventionally treated mainly with synthetics to suppress these symptoms this, however, causes additional other health issues.

To answer this vicious cycle with power of nature, we may focus on following ...

NATURAL THERAPIES – SCIENTIFICALLY VERIFIED

Such as ...

Diet

Based on the fact that MS is causing inflammation, science – with special reference to *Johns Hopkins University* in Baltimore, MD – recommends for MS patients to consume primarily low fat and high fiber diet, as you find it in fruits, vegetables, and whole grains.

With special reference to
- Vitamins (A/B-12/C/E)
to fight, inter alia, *inflammation* and *urinary tract infection*
and
- Calcium
to avoid, inter alia, *osteoporosis.*

Vice-versa, MS patients may refrain from saturated fat, high fat dairy, and salt.

Herbs

According to research at, inter alia, the *University of Colorado* in Denver, CO, and verified by the U.S. *National Center for Complementary and Integrative Health (NIH),* following herbs may be beneficial for MS patients, as follows.

- *Echinacea*

As it may support the immune system of MS patients.

- *Valerian root*

to thwart, inter alia, fatigue.

- *St. John's Wort*

To counteract depression naturally.

- *Cranberry*

To help with pain and spasticity, as well as urinary tract infection.

Exercise

In order to stay strong and active, when affected by MS, the *University of Pennsylvania* in Philadelphia, PA, recommends physical exercise.

IN A NUTSHELL

Multiple Sclerosis (MS) is a damage to the central nervous system caused by attack of our own immune system. Leading to different health issues which have not been solved conventionally yet. That's why we focus on medicinal answers from nature's kingdom in this chapter.

29. CUT CHOLESTEROL WITH HEALTHY DRINKS?

THE PHILOSOPHY BEHIND

Cholesterol is an important substance our body basically needs to establish and support cells and hormones. Consisting of 2 parts: 'good' high-density lipoprotein (HDL) and 'bad' low-density lipoprotein (LDL). It is vital for our health to keep both in a balanced relationship in favor of an appropriate amount of good HDL. With special reference to our heart and cardiovascular system. Unfortunately yet, this relationship is highly out of control in our industrialized society. Primarily due to unhealthy diet. Fortunately, nature offers us some nutrition to balance out this disparity in favor of our health.

Including

HEALTHY DRINKS – SCIENTIFICALLY VALIDATED

E.g.,

Green tea

Based on its natural constituents *catechins* and *epigallocatechin gallate*, green tea may lower 'bad' LDL cholesterol.

According to research at the *Government College University Faisalabad* in Faisalabad, Pakistan, these natural constituents of green tea may lower total cholesterol and cut LDL cholesterol specifically by more than 30%.

Similar the situation with

Tomato juice

because of its compound *lycopene* as well as its content of *niacin* (vitamin B-3) and *fiber*.

With respect to total cholesterol and reducing the amount of 'bad' LDL.

Based on research at, inter alia, *China Medical University* in Taichung, Taiwan.

Oat milk

According to research at, inter alia,
- *Universite d'Auvergne* in Clermont-Ferrand, France
  and the
- *University of Ottawa* in Ottawa, Canada

the substance *beta-glucan* in oats helps to cut down cholesterol absorption, reducing LDL specifically.

Similar the effect of

Soy milk

According to *Heart UK – The Cholesterol Charity* in Maidenhead, UK, to reduce and manage cholesterol.

Plant-based milk smoothies

Both, oat and soy milk you may also combine to a smoothie by adding per cup of 250 ml additionally cholesterol-lowering vegetables and/or fruits like, inter alia,
- 2/3 cup pumpkin puree
- 1 cup of Swiss chard/kale
- 1 slice of melon or mango
- 1 banana
- 2 small plums
- 1 handful of prunes or grapes

Based on research at, inter alia, *McGill University* in Sainte-Anne-de-Bellevue, Canada.

Berry smoothies

This is another helpful smoothy for cholesterol management because of berries' content of fiber and antioxidants. Specifically the antioxidant anthocyanins as you find it, inter alia, in
- blueberries
- strawberries
- raspberries
- blackberries

According to research at, inter alia, *George Mason University* in Fairfax, VA.

Cocoa drink

As you may know, cocoa is the main part of dark chocolate. Thereby, its antioxidants of *flavanols* are very helpful in cholesterol management in both directions:
- increasing 'good' HDL
  and
- reducing 'bad' LDL

According to research at, inter alia,
- *University of Reading* in Reading, UK
  and
- *University Düsseldorf* in Düsseldorf, Germany

Now, as we know which drinks to prefer for appropriate cholesterol management, we shall briefly focus on

DRINKS TO AVOID

according to the *American Heart Association.*

These are basically drinks
- high in saturated fats
  and those
- high in sugar adding up to more than 12 ounces per day.

Drinks high in saturated fats

Inter alia,
- coffee/tea with, e.g., high fat milk or cream
- ice-cream based drinks
- pressed coconut drinks
- drinks/smoothies with coconut/palm oils
- products of high fat milk

Sugary drinks

Inter alia,
- energy drinks
- fruit juices
- soda/pop
- sweetened coffee/tea
- (hot) chocolate
- sweetened milk products
- sports drink

- prepackaged smoothies

IN A NUTSHELL

While cholesterol is basically a vital substance for our health, its appropriate level and relationship between 'good' (HDL) & 'bad' (LDL) cholesterol is of importance. With special reference to our heart and cardiovascular system. Since an unhealthy level of cholesterol may cause, inter alia, even stroke and heart attack. In order to be on the safe side, the American Heart Association (AHA) recommends certain natural drinks we are focusing on in this chapter. Scientifically verified by U.S. & international medical science.

30. DIABETES: GI – THE MAGIC FORMULA

THE PHILOSOPHY BEHIND

Diabetes is one of the most debilitating diseases in our industrialized society with high mortality rate. Fortunately, both is manageable – based on laws of nature. With special reference to the glycemic index (GI) in our foods being substantially responsible for the sugar content in our blood circulation.

The *International Organization for Standardization (ISO)* classifies the GI content in our foods on a scale from 1 to 100. I.e., a GI of
- 55 or less means *low*
- 56-69 means *medium*
- 70 or more means *high*

Verified by the *American Diabetes Association.*

According to the U.S. *Glycemic Index Foundation (GIF),* foods with low GI factor help to prevent and manage diabetes (and other health issues - as mentioned in following).

Scientifically verified internationally by, inter alia,
- *University of Greenwich* in London, UK
- *Federal University of Technology* in Akure, Nigeria
- *Soochow University* in Suzhou, China
- *Huazhong University of Science and Technology* in Wuhan, China
- *University of Canberra* in Canberra, Australia

Including *gestational diabetes,* i.e. diabetes during the time of pregnancy.

As scientifically supported by, inter alia, *Changzhou Jintan People's Hospital* in Changzhou, China.

Additional health benefits

According to the U.S. *Glycemic Index Foundation,* a low GI may be helpful also for other health issues.

E.g.

- *weight management*

according to research at, inter alia, *Universitat Rovira i Virgili* in Reus, Spain, and the *Fred Hutchinson Cancer Research Center* in Seattle, WA.

As well as

- *depression*
- *fatigue*
  and
- *inertia*

according to research at *Fred Hutchinson Cancer Research Center*.

Also, the GI is of high relevance when it comes to

- *cancer*

as based on meta-analysis by, inter alia,
- *Universita degli Studi di Milano* in Milano, Italy
- *St. Michael's Hospital* in Toronto, Canada
- *Instituto Nazionale Tumori* in Naples, Italy

Not to forget about cardiovascular disease with special reference to

- *coronary heart disease*

according to another meta-analysis at *Independent Nutrition Logic* in Wymondham, UK

Therefore, the GI factor is especially of relevance when it comes to our daily nutrition. I.e. foods containing a certain amount of GI with its effect on blood sugar.

Doing justice accordingly, appreciate following highly reputable international findings about

LOW GI MEAL OPTIONS – SCIENTIFICALLY VALIDATED

As verified by the U.S. *Centers for Disease Control and Prevention,* based on research at, inter alia,
- *University of Toronto* in Toronto, Canada
- *Harvard School of Public Health* in Boston, MA
- *University of Saskatchewan* in Saskatoon, Canada

- *Lund University* in Lund, Sweden
- *University of Sydney* in Sydney, Australia
- *University of Parma* in Parma, Italy
- *University of Bonn* in Bonn, Germany
- *Universita degli Studi di Milano* in Milano, Italy
- *Brown University* in Providence, RI
- *University of Copenhagen* in Copenhagen, Denmark
- *Federico II University* in Naples, Italy
- *University Pierre et Marie Curie* in Paris, France
- *University of Athens Medical School* in Athens, Greece

With additional relevance of fiber and whole grains, according to research at, inter alia,

- *Arizona State University* in Phoenix, AZ
- *University of Otago* in Dunedin, New Zealand
- *University of Minnesota* in St. Paul, MN

Based on this scientific background, see a recommended potential daily low GI meal plan as follows:

- **Breakfast**

  - buckwheat pancakes with berries
  - scrambled eggs with smoked salmon
  - breakfast quesadillas with spinach/black beans/mushrooms

- **Lunch**

  - black bean/cauliflower/celeriac soup
  - mango chicken & almond on rye bread

- **Dinner**

  - Indian-style spiced vegetable
  - lamb shanks with barley/garden peas/mint
  - Tex-Mex tofu soft tacos

- **Snacks**

  - homemade full-of-fruit muffins
  - roasted soy nuts
  - slice of cinnamon/almond/oat loaf

Vice-versa, be careful about *high* GI foods with reference to the *International Tables of Glycemic Index and Glycemic Load Values*, according to the *American Diabetes Association*.

Such as, inter alia,
- white and whole wheat bread
- breakfast cereals/cereal bars
- white rice
- potatoes & fries
- chips & rice crackers
- cakes/cookies/sweat treats
- dried fruits like dates/raisins/cranberries
- fruits like watermelon & pineapple
- sweetened dairy products like fruit yogurts

IN A NUTSHELL

High blood sugar based on high glycemic foods is a crucial point behind diabetes and other debilitating diseases. To manage naturally, it is of high relevance to understand which foods have a low glycemic index (GI) and which do not. Find scientifically verified answers on international basis in this chapter.

31. LONGEVITY DEPENDING ON WHAT?

THE PHILOSOPHY BEHIND

As you know from our previous publications and seminars, longevity is basically a matter of manageable lifestyle. With special reference to healthy diet and physical exercise. Unfortunately, however, most of our citizens do not follow this prerequisite.

Not only...

Walk off mortality?

According to scientific study at *Inje University* in Gyeongsangnam-do, Republic of Korea, with prospects over 85 years old, demonstrated that walking at least for one hour per week may well cut down the risk of all-cause mortality, cardiovascular and diabetes related specifically.

Even more, as there are ...

ADDITIONAL FACTORS – SCIENTIFICALLY VERIFIED

As we learn from research at the *Ecole Polytechnique Federale de Lausanne* in Lausanne, Switzerland, additional to our self-chosen basic pillars of lifestyle other – and partly less manageable – certain factors play a role in terms of longevity.

With special reference to

Age & Gender

Scientifically verified by the *Institute of Prevention and Clinical Medicine* in Bratislava, Slovakia, women live longer than men, if they are practicing physically. Independent of their respective genes.

In figures, in the U.S. life expectancy of women, in average, is 79 years in this case, to be compared with 73 years of men. As confirmed by U.S. governmental Centers for Disease Control and Prevention (CDC).

Even more, there are different factors to disfavor men when it comes to life extension such as, inter alia:

- Women tend less likely to suicide than men
  (based on research at *Washington University School of Medicine* in St. Louis, MO)
- Men are visiting a doctor less frequent than women
  (according to research at, inter alia, the *University of Melbourne* in Melbourne, Australia and the *University of Glasgow* in Glasgow, UK)
- Risk of occupational injuries & death is higher in men than women

Although women are more predisposed to debilitating diseases such as, inter alia,

- Depression
  (according to findings at the *Ottawa Hospital Research Institute* in Ottawa, Canada)
- Stroke
  (according to the American Stroke Association)
- Alzheimer's disease
  (according to research at the *University of Pennsylvania* in University Park, PA)

IN A NUTSHELL

While longevity is basically an issue of 2 manageable pillars - healthy diet and physical exercise - there are additional factors with special reference to lifestyle and health you need to understand in order to manage them as far as possible in order to extend your lifespan.

32. WHICH FOODS HELP LOSING WEIGHT?

THE PHILOSOPHY BEHIND

Although the U.S. is spending most for conventional medicine per capita worldwide, some 80% of health issues and non-age-related deaths are primarily the consequence of unnatural lifestyle. With two thirds of the adult population being overweight and half of those obese, as one of the leading causes behind. Based on the fact that our body is a strongly interrelated and complex biologic-ecologic phenomenon. In line with laws of nature. That's why body weight has a considerable impact on our health.

However, unlike manifold assumptions, losing weight is primarily not an issue of food *quantity*. Since cutting calories may not only give the feeling of hunger and deprivation, reducing food consumption may also have a negative impact on our health in general. What really counts in this case, is the *quality* of certain nutrients found in specific foods we need for our health and for regulating our weight at the same time. The *American Diabetes Association (ADA)* has listed these basic nutrients as follows.

- **Vitamins**

    - A/C/E/K
      and
    - B (with special reference to B-1 Thiamin/B-2 Riboflavin/B-3 Niacin/B-12 Cobalamin)

Also

- **Minerals**

    like

    - magnesium
    - calcium
    - zinc
      and
    - iron

As well as

- ***Antioxidants***

To ward off damage from so called free radicals which support chronic diseases. In this context, especially relevant antioxidants are, inter alia, vitamins A/C/E and selenium.

Additionally,

- ***Healthy fats***

With special reference to omega-3e fatty acids and monounsaturated fat. Relevant for, inter alia, heart health and hormone regulation.

And

- ***Fiber***

As the non-digestible constituents of *carbohydrates*, to be found in
- fruits
- vegetables
- whole grains

Not only giving us a feeling of fullness but also helping with, inter alia, bowel regulation and cholesterol management.

Finally

- ***Phytonutrients***

I.e. those pigments giving fruits and vegetables their specific color.

Leaves us with the question in which...

TYPES OF FOODS – SCIENTIFICALLY VERIFIED

...we find these nutrients best?

In fact, there is no specific single food representing all relevant constituents our body needs for health – and appropriate weight.

Doing justice accordingly, not only has the *American Diabetes Association (ADA)* listed nutrients for healthy weight. According to the U.S. *Centers for Disease Control and Prevention (CDC)*, following 'super foods' – containing these nutrients - are recommended to support our health and control our weight.

Scientifically verified, inter alia, at *Louisiana State University* in Baton Rouge, LA, and the *University of Laval* in Quebec City, Canada.

These foods are, inter alia...

- **Fruits**

such as

  - Berries (especially blueberries)

because of their content of *vitamins C & K*, also *potassium* and *manganese*, as well as *fiber*.

And

  - Citrus fruits (like lemons/oranges/grapefruit)

containing, inter alia, *potassium, vitamin C, folate* and *fiber*.

- **Vegetables**

Such as

  - dark green leafy vegetables (like kale/spinach/collards)

because of inherent *vitamins A/C/E/K* and *minerals calcium/potassium/iron*.

Also

  - sweet potatoes

as an excellent source of *vitamins A & C*, as well as *fiber* and *potassium*.

- **Beans**

like kidney/pinto/navy beans.

Containing, inter alia, minerals *magnesium & potassium, fiber,* and *protein* like meat.

- **Whole grains**

like whole grain barley/whole oatmeal/quinoa.

With the content of *B vitamins,* minerals such as *magnesium, chromium* and *iron.* Also *fiber* and *folate.*

- **Nuts/seeds**

With special reference to flaxseeds and walnuts.

As an excellent source of *omega-3 fatty acids* which we find also in

- **Fish**

Such as salmon, herring, trout and albacore tuna.

- **Milk**

containing *vitamin D* and *calcium.*

Thereby,

- **Yogurt**

comes with the special benefit of supporting loss of body fat, cutting food intake and promotes feeling of fullness.

Additionally, *CDC* recommends

- **Poultry**
  and
- **Lean meat**

but at the same time warns of foods high in sugar, salt and saturated fat.

How include these 'super foods' in your daily diet?

Besides consuming some of these as a snack and/or dessert, adjust your regular nutrition to most healthy *Mediterranean diet* which covers many of the aforementioned 'super foods'.

With the benefit that Mediterranean diet may well prevent obesity, according to research at, inter alia, the *University of Bologna* in Bologna, Italy.

COMPLEMENTARY HEALTH BENEFITS

Scientifically verified at, inter alia, the *University of Mauritius* in Reduit, Mauritius, these are

- ***Fruits & vegetables***

protecting also against *diabetes* and *cancer*.

- ***Fiber***

on the other hand, additionally to promoting the feeling of fullness, also may help against *inflammation*, based on research at, inter alia, the *University of Warwick* and *Coventry University* – both in Coventry, UK – and *Charite University* in Berlin, Germany.

- ***Antioxidant foods***

According to, inter alia, the U.S. *Academy of Nutrition and Dietetics* (founded 1917 in Cleveland, OH), foods rich in antioxidants are beneficial in cases of *heart disease* and certain types of *cancer*.

- ***Omega-3 fat foods***

are helpful in cases of *heart disease* and in supporting the *immune system*.

According to the U.S. *National Institute of Health (NIH)*.

IN A NUTSHELL

Appropriate diet, besides physical exercise, is one of the vital pillars our health and body weight is resting on. In terms of certain nutrients we find in specific foods. As recommended, inter alia, by the U.S. *Centers for Disease Control and Prevention (CDC)*, scientifically verified.

33. TRAIN YOUR BRAIN FOR MENTAL POWER

THE PHILOSOPHY BEHIND

As you know, and as you have learned also from our previous publications, our body is a very complex biologic-ecologic phenomenon. Physically, and mentally. In fact, our brain as the most complex part of our body, is the control center and switch board for regulating our bodily functions, and our lifestyle activities. With special reference to our memory, creativity and intelligence. This comprehensively overriding responsibility requires to take care of it, accordingly.

BRAIN-RELATED ACTIONS – SCIENTIFICALLY VERIFIED

While our brain is challenged every day in one or another way automatically with respect to our lifestyle, we can additionally support its power with certain natural actions. Not only for better performance per se but also to relieve age-related degeneration.

Just to list a sample of 20 actions in following.

Sport activities

Basically, sport activities are challenging physically and mentally, with respect to
- multitasking
- planning
- sustained attention
- skill adapting rapidly to changed situations

With special reference to the fact that athletes of this kind are improving their attention and the speed of processing information.

According to international research at, inter alia,
- *Autonomous University of Nuevo Leon* in San Nicolas de los Garza, Mexico
- *University of Malaga* in Malaga, Spain
- *Western Norway University of Applied Sciences & University of Bergen* (both in Bergen, Norway)

Physical exercise

However, even if you do not practice a specific type of sport, just physical exercise on a regular basis is helpful for both – mind and body. As it will improve your

- memory
- cognition
  and
- motor coordination

Based on research at, inter alia, *Inha University School of Medicine* in Incheon, South Korea.

Dancing

Not to forget that also dancing is a type of physical exercise with benefit for our cognitive power, such as

- memory
- organization
  and
- planning

with special reference to rhythm and balance.

According to the U.S. *Centers for Disease Control and Prevention (CDC).*

Socializing

Meeting frequently with friends is mentally engaging and may avoid cognitive decline and dementia.

With special reference to, inter alia,

- playing games
- having discussions
  or
- engage in sports

According to a 28-year follow-up meta-analysis at the *University College London* in London, UK.

Playing card games

To play card games is not only a funny way of socializing but also decreases the risk of cognitive impairment especially in cases of older adults.

In cases of memory card games this has an impact also on short-term memory.

According to a meta-analysis at *Mayo Clinic* in Rochester, MN & Scottsdale, AZ.

Playing chess

To play chess is an excellent cognitive modality to support and improve
- memory
- information processing speed
  and
- executive functioning to adapt and monitor in order to meet goals set

According to a meta-analysis at, inter alia, the *University of Nottingham* in Nottingham, UK.

Playing video games

Puzzle/strategy/action video games may well help with improvements in
- problem solving
- attention
  and
- cognitive flexibility

Based on research at, inter alia, the *University of Wisconsin* in Madison, WI.

Meditation

Meditation – involving to focus attention in a controlled and calm way – not only may improve brain's power to process information but also to slow down brain aging.

According to the U.S. *National Center for Complementary and Integrative Health (NIH).*

Tai chi practice

This type of physical exercise, originating in China, is a most effective one for mind and body alike. It comes with rhythmic breathing, gentle body movements and also meditation. Enhancing connectivity between certain parts of the brain. On one side improving cognition, and on the other, cutting down rate of memory loss.

Based on research at, inter alia, *Beihang University* in China's capital Beijing.

Visualizing

This way, a mental image of certain information may be formed as a kind of picture or animated scene in order to organize the information better and to come up with the right decision.

To be done in order to imagine expected scenes vividly ahead and in detail.

Supported by research at, inter alia, the *University of Utah* in Salt Lake City, UT, and the *University of California-Santa Barbara* in Santa Barbara, CA.

Jigsaw puzzles

To complete a jigsaw puzzle may not only help passing the time, but support brain activity at the same time.

Just as puzzles activate certain cognitive functions like, inter alia,
- working memory
- mental rotation
- reasoning
- perception

which may also relieve brain aging.

Based on research at, inter alia,
- *Ulm University* in Ulm
  &
- *University of Hohenheim* in Stuttgart
  (both Germany)
  as well as the Spanish
- *Universidad Nacional de Educacion a Distancia (UNED)*

Crossword puzzles

Also these kinds of puzzles stimulate the brain by delaying the onset of memory decline. With special reference to preclinical dementia.

Based on research at, inter alia,
- *University of California & VA Medical Center*
  (both in San Diego, CA)
- *Albert Einstein College of Medicine* in Bronx, NY
  &

- *Mayo Clinic* in Jacksonville, FL

Playing sudoku

This type of number puzzle may support cognitive function especially of adults beyond age 50.

According to research at, inter alia, the *University of Exeter* in Exeter, UK.

Playing checkers

Practicing stimulating games like this may lead to improvement of markers of cognitive health especially in cases where risk of Alzheimer's disease is relevant.

Based on research at, inter alia, the *University of Wisconsin School of Medicine and Public Health* in Madison, WI.

Learning new skills

To acquire additional and cognitively strengthening skills like, e.g., photography or quilting, etc., may support brain function with special reference to our memory. Especially later in years.

According to research at, inter alia, the *University of Texas at Dallas* in Richardson, TX.

Bilingualism

To learn and speak a new (second) language supports connectivity between certain brain areas which may well reduce the risk of dementia like Alzheimer's.

Based on research at, inter alia, *Konyang University* in Daejeon, South Korea.

New hobbies

To create a new hobby can well support mental capacity. Especially, as motor skills can be activated with following types of hobbies:
- drawing
- painting
- embroidery
- dancing
- knitting

Same applies to...

Learning a musical instrument

... as this may support the power of coordination in the brain. Not only for young people but also for elders with an aging brain.

According to research at, inter alia, the *University of California* in Los Angeles, CA.

Listening to music

In general, listening to enjoyable music connects different parts in the brain leading not only to better cognitive function but to well-being in an overall way.

Based on international research at, inter alia, the *University of Leuven* in Leuven, Belgium, and *Aarhus University* in Aarhus, Denmark.

Sleeping

Although to sleep doesn't sound like a type of 'action', yes, sleep is well an important issue for both – body and mind. As it is not only relaxing us physically but also, inter alia,

- reduces mental fatigue
- boosts memory recall
  and
- regulates metabolism

According to international research at, inter alia, *Mayo Clinic* in Rochester, MN, and the *Medical University of Lublin* in Lublin, Poland.

IN A NUTSHELL

Our brain is the most important and complex part of our body. As it is the control center and switch board for regulating not only our bodily functions, but our lifestyle activities in general. Fortunately, nature leads us the way how to support our brain's power with specific actions. In this blog you learn about a sample of 20 of these powerful and easy to follow actions.

34. HOW SUPPORT HEALTH AT HOME OFFICE?

THE PHILOSOPHY BEHIND

To work from home is all but new for many businesses and job descriptions. However, it has entered the forefront in many work relations during COVID-19 pandemic, and more companies than before continue offering it to their employees.

However, while this comes with certain economic benefits (e.g. in order not to lose the job at all), there are also drawbacks for our health involved – physically, mentally, and socially. Based on the fact that any lifestyle factor comes with an impact on our well-being in general. Geographic disposition of workplace being no exception.

Fortunately, there are ...

HEALTH-RELATED ACTIONS – SCIENTIFICALLY VALIDATED

... in order to support our wellness, without harming business.

Like the following.

Work-life balance

In fact, the limits between work and private life can get well mixed up especially at a home office. Temporally, and spatially. With well a detriment for health.

Accordingly, the *American Health Information Management Association (AHIMA)* recommends to set up a daily work schedule. Including not only specific time for lunch but also a 15-minute break in the morning and a 15-minute break in the afternoon. Plus time for relaxation at the end of workday.

Scientifically validated also at the *Simon Fraser University* in Vancouver, Canada.

Daily routine

Thereby, the U.S. *Centers for Disease Control and Prevention (CDC)* recommend to implant a daily routine in time of private life off work which may reduce the risk of stress.

E.g., by sticking to the same daily times when to get up in the morning and when to go to bed. Appreciating that 7 hours of sleep regularly are advisable health-wise.

Mindfulness

Based on research at, inter alia, *Simon Fraser University* in Vancouver, Canada, mindfulness is another way to reduce stress when working from home. As it helps to observe experiences, but without need of judgment directly. Thus increasing objectivity.

Healthy diet

According to the U.S. *National Heart, Lung, and Blood Institute (NHLBI)*, and verified by the U.S. *Centers for Disease Control and Prevention (CDC)*, following a healthy eating plan is especially recommended at home offices with more freedom than at workplace. With the danger of skipping meals more likely in this case.

Thereby, the healthy eating plan (with controlled portion sizes) may emphasize
- fruits
- vegetables
- whole grains
- fat-free/low-fat dairy products

and also include
- lean meats
- poultry
- fish
- beans
- eggs
- nuts

but, on the other hand, may limit
- saturated/trans fats
- sodium
- added sugar

Staying hydrated

According to *CDC*, it is also important to stay hydrated at the home office, in order to avoid constipation and mood swings. Preferably with water, and potentially in addition with coffee and tea. Not sugary liquids like energy drinks/sodas/fruit drinks.

Regular exercise

At the same time, the U.S. *Department of Homeland Security (DHS)* recommends to counterbalance the physical activity of commuting to/from workplace by implanting either/or/and brisk walk or exercise with fitness video or mobile app during workday at the home office. Potentially along with some pushups.

Also may a standing desk be in favor, instead of a sitting desk.

In order to avoid physical inactivity at the home office.

Posture comfort

CDC recommends to organize the home office in a way to allow best posture and to avoid back pain.

By help of an office chair with armrests and high enough to allow feet resting on the floor flat. And with officer's hips and knees being slightly above 90-degree angle. Also supporting curvature of lower back.

Thereby, the computer monitor may be away an arm's length, with the monitor's top being either at or below the eye level.

Socializing

Unlike at common workplaces, to connect with colleagues and other persons related to work is difficult – but important also mentally. In order to avoid loneliness.

The more important it is to enter conversations at least electronically even with people who are not related workwise and who may be located out of physical reach.

According to research at, inter alia,
- *Curtin University* in Perth, Australia
- *Beijing Normal University* in China's capital Beijing and
- *Shanghai University* in Shanghai, China

IN A NUTSHELL

In order to avoid (or at least reduce the risk of) infection with the COVID-19 virus by contracting and/or spreading it, home office has become the alternative of outsourced workplace in many cases. However, with some negative impact on our physical, mental, and social well-being. This can be encountered with health-related actions, as scientifically verified.

35. SAVE YOUR HEART WITH CHOLESTEROL?

THE PHILOSOPHY BEHIND

The U.S. is foremost in conventional medicine worldwide, with – inter alia -

- 1st open heart surgery (Dr. Michael E. DeBakey)
- 1st Artificial heart transplant (Dr. Denton Cooley)
- 1st heart repair w/stem cells (Dr. Ed Marban)
- 1st modern cardiologist (Dr. Paul Dudley White – personal physician of President Eisenhower)

Still – according to statistics of the *World Health Organization (WHO)* – more than 80% of non-age-related premature deaths are the consequence of unsolved ('chronic') health issues. With heart failure on top of the list. As confirmed also by the U.S. governmental *Centers for Disease Control and Prevention (CDC)*.

One of the major causes behind of this mostly preventable vicious cycle of heart-related mortality is cholesterol - ?

Basically, cholesterol is a profound module for our health and existence. As it is organically produced as a natural waxy and fat-like substance by an enzyme in our body naturally to support healthy cell membranes and to produce bile for detoxifying our body.

Composed of high-density lipoprotein/HDL (so called 'good' cholesterol) and low-density lipoprotein/LDL ('bad cholesterol'). However, while 'bad' cholesterol our body does not need for its regular functioning, it endangers our heart. Other than HDL which delivers LDL to the liver to be removed from the body. In fact, a heart attack is signaling too high total cholesterol in the blood and lack of healthy balance between HDL/LDL.

In statistical terms: going by the fact that heart failure potentially leading to premature mortality comes usually later in life, recommended limits for adults are, according to the U.S. governmental *National Heart, Lung, and Blood Institute*:
- Total cholesterol less than 200 mg/dl
- LDL ('bad' cholesterol) less than 100 mg/dl
- HDL ('good' cholesterol) higher than 60 mg/dl

Disregarding and even violating these limits, potentially leading to heart-related mortality in many cases, is significantly caused by unhealthy diet. With special reference to high levels of saturated and trans fats (like cheese, eggs and meat), and which can clog arteries. Enhancing the risk of heart disease, peripheral artery disease and stroke.

CHOLESTEROL-FRIENDLY FOODS – SCIENTIFICALLY VALIDATED

Fortunately yet, there are many types of natural foods to manage cholesterol for healthy and long life. (In favor of more HDL and less LDL, still keeping total and LDL cholesterol low.) Inter alia,...

- *Apples*

According to research at, inter alia,
- *University of Reading* in Reading, UK
&
- *Fondazione Edmund Mach* in San Michele all'Adige, Italy,
2 apples a day may well decrease not only total cholesterol but LDL in particular. Based on the fact that in average, one apple may include 3-7 grams of dietary fiber.

- *Broccoli*

As a cruciferous green leafy (cruciferous) vegetable may prevent heart disease by lowering artery-blocking cholesterol in blood.

According to research at, inter alia, *Vanderbilt University School of Medicine* in Nashville, TN. Scientifically verified also at the *Western Regional Research Center* of USDA-ARS in Albany, New York.

- *Eggplants*

Based on its high content of fiber, these vegetables are not only beneficial for managing cholesterol but they also cut down the risk of heart disease and stroke.

According to the *American Heart Association (AHA)*.

- *Okra*

("lady's fingers" – as folk saying goes) can help lowering cholesterol because of the gel *mucilage* it contains and which also helps cholesterol leaving our body through stool.

Based on research at *Wollega University* in Addis Ababa, Ethiopia.

Similar

- *Legumes/pulses*

like peas/lentils/beans/chickpeas not only can lower the heart-harming LDL cholesterol, their contents of, inter alia, protein, fiber and antioxidant polyphenols are beneficial for health in general and heart health in particular.

Based on research at, inter alia, the *University of Toronto* and *St. Michael's Hospital,* both in Toronto, Canada.

In more detail:

Dry Beans

like black beans, navy beans and kidney beans, being very high in plant proteins and fiber, as well as minerals and vitamin B-complex, can decrease cholesterol. According to scientific findings at, inter alia, *St. Michael's Hospital* in Toronto, Canada.

Soybeans

just as related products like soy yogurt/soy milk/tofu have cholesterol-lowering power, as soy protein can reduce LDL cholesterol considerably just by intake of 25 grams of soy protein daily over 6 weeks.

Scientifically verified at, inter alia, the *University of Toronto* in Toronto, Canada.

Lentils

because of its very high fiber content. Based on research at *Pennsylvania State University* and the *University of South Australia* in Adelaide.

According to research at *Shahid Beheshti University of Medical Sciences* in Tehran & *Tabriz University of Medical Sciences* in Tabriz, Iran, lentils cut down 'bad' LDL cholesterol by more than 10%.

In this context we may also see

- *Oats*

Because of its high content of soluble fiber in oats for cholesterol management. Additional to its cardiovascular benefit.

Based on research at, inter alia, the *University of Kentucky* in Lexington, KY, and the *City University of New York*.

According to the *National Diabetes, Obesity, and Cholesterol Foundation (N-DOC)* in New Delhi, India, consuming 70 grams of oats per day may decrease LDL cholesterol by more than 10% per month.

Another grain rich in dietary fiber (with special reference to beta-glucan, as in oats) and of relevance for cutting down LDL cholesterol is

- *Barley*

Additional to the fact that barley is benefitting the heart in general.

As based on research at, inter alia, the
- *University of Louisville* in Louisville, KY
- *The Czech Academy of Sciences* in Prague, Czech Republic and the
- *University of Ottawa* in Canada's capital Ottawa

Boiled

- *Kale*

is another excellent candidate of nature's family, with just one cup containing almost 5 grams of dietary fiber, lowering total cholesterol and especially LDL.

Additionally, since kale is also rich in antioxidants, it is of great benefit for the heart.

Based on research at, inter alia, the *University of Warwick* in Coventry, UK.

- *Olive oil*

Extra virgin olive oil as a source of monounsaturated fatty acids – with special reference to the heart-healthy Mediterranean diet - may well relieve inflammation und reduce LDL ('bad') cholesterol by enhancing HDL ('good') cholesterol. Besides of its cardiovascular benefit.

Based on research at, inter alia, *Institut Municipal d'Investigacio Medica (IMIM)* in Barcelona, Spain, and the *Instituto Superiore di Sanita* in Rome, Italy.

- *Nuts*

As nuts (like pistachios /almonds/pecans/hazelnuts/walnuts/Brazil nuts/cashews) are not only rich in vitamins/minerals/fiber/protein/ antioxidants but also in unsaturated fats.

With the benefit of cutting down LDL cholesterol, especially when replacing saturated fats in diet. Additionally, they are rich in fiber to ward off cholesterol and help to excrete it from our body.

Additionally to the fact that (all) nuts are basically beneficial for heart health.

According to, inter alia, the *American Heart Association.*

Just let's focus on 2 different types in more detail as scientifically verified: almonds and walnuts:

Almonds

 containing B & E vitamins as well as minerals. According to renowned *Linus Pauling Institute* in Oregon, named after 2 times Nobel Prize laureate in medicine and founder of Orthomolecular Medicine, Dr. Linus Pauling.

Scientifically verified also at *Tufts University* in Boston, MA.

Walnuts

being rich in omegoa-3 fatty acids, not only improve blood vessel function but reduce inflammation as well. According to research at, inter alia, *Loma Linda University* in Loma Linda, California, and *Harvard University* in Boston, MA.

Even more. Based on a meta-analysis of 26 clinical trials, consuming walnuts regularly can may reduce total cholesterol by 3.25% and 'bad' LDL cholesterol by 3.73%, according to the *American Society for Nutrition* in Rockville, MD

In general, according to research at *Pennsylvania State University* in Philadelphia, PA, and the *University of Guelph* in Guelph, Canada, nuts can reduce cholesterol in blood by 6%.

Another most valuable natural food to reduce 'bad' (LDL) cholesterol - without lowering the 'good' HDL cholesterol - are

- *Avocados*

Not only this. Since avocados are loaded with heart-healthy nutrients, with special reference to monounsaturated fats (in fact, one cup/150 grams of avocados contain almost 15 grams of monounsaturated fats), they also reduce the risk of heart disease and stroke considerably.
According to research at, inter alia, *Pennsylvania State University* in University Park, PA, and the *University of South Australia* in Adelaide, Australia.

- *Fish*

As a rich source of omega-3 fats like salmon/sardines/mackerel it may support HDL's activity in the body by reducing the formation of cholesterol crystals in the arteries.

With special reference to the omega-3 type *eicosapentaenoic acid (EPA)* which also reduces level of triglycerides (a fat entering the blood after meal), preventing atherosclerosis. Accordingly, it is very beneficial for our heart in general.

Based on research at, inter alia, *Harvard Medical School* in Boston, MA.

Also

- *Orange Juice*

rich in potassium and magnesium, as well as vitamins A, C and B-complex, proven to reduce cholesterol. According to, inter alia, The U.S. *Department of Agriculture*, as well as *Health and Human Services*.

On the other hand, when drinking 3 eight-ounce glasses of (unsweetened)

- *Cranberry juice*

per day may raise the 'good' HDL cholesterol in blood by 10% - thus reducing heart disease risk by some 40%.

Based on research at, inter alia, the *University of Sranton* in Sranton, PA.

Also, a study from the *Islamic Azad University* in Tehran and *Isfahan University of Medical Sciences* in Isfahan – both Iran – recommends

- *Balsamic vinegar*

for a variety of health benefits (such as improving skin health, promoting healthy digestion, reducing blood sugar and blood pressure, losing weight, treating wounds and relieving congestion) – but also for *lowering cholesterol.*

IN A NUTSHELL

Cholesterol, being blamed responsible for heart disease with premature death in many cases, has got 2 seemingly 'schizophrenic' characteristics: HDL ('good' cholesterol) to support healthy cell membranes and to produce bile for detoxifying our body. As well as LDL ('bad' cholesterol) endangering our heart with blockage of the arteries leading potentially to stroke. Fortunately yet, nature offers us nutrition-related ways out of this vicious cycle. Scientifically validated.

36. SUFFER ANXIETY? ADJUST YOUR LIFESTYLE!

THE PHILOSOPHY BEHIND

Anxiety is one of the most prevalent problems of mental health in our society. With almost 20% of U.S. adult citizens affected. Along with symptoms like tension, nervousness, chest pain and a racing heart – etc.

Since, in most cases, it is related to stressful situations, handling both is certainly of relevance. Preferably naturally, not with synthetics. E.g. with herbs, as you have learned from our previous publications.

LIFESTYLE ADJUSTMENTS – SCIENTIFICALLY VERIFIED

Even more, you may adjust your daily lifestyle with certain modalities to relieve anxiety. Self-administrated, without sophisticated therapy.

Just to pick a few examples...

Physical exercise

This, according to *Duke University Medical Center* in Durham, NC. has not only physical but also mental benefits. Relieving anxiety being no exception.

Such as a brisk walk of only 30 minutes having already a positive impact on depression and anxiety.

Supported by research at, inter alia,
- *University of Texas* in Austin, TX
- *University of Texas MD Anderson Cancer Center* in Houston, TX
- *University of Houston* in Houston, TX
- *Southern Methodist University* in Dallas, TX
- *University of California* in San Diego, CA
- *San Francisco VA Medical Center* in San Francisco, CA
- *Louisiana State University* in Baton Rouge, LA
- *Boston University* in Boston, MA
- *Howard University in Washington, D.C.*

Scientifically verified by the *U.S. Centers for Disease Control and Prevention.*

Meditation

Slowing down racing thoughts, meditation may help to manage anxiety (and stress). With special reference to mindfulness.

Based on research at, inter alia, *Boston University* in Boston, MA, and *Indira Gandhi Government Medical College* in Nagpur, India.

Companionship with pets

Pets (like dogs, cats & other small mammals) are well known for offering help with mental issues, anxiety included.

Based on research at, inter alia,
- *Purdue University* in West Lafayette, IN
- *University of Manchester* in Manchester, UK
- *Universita degli Studi di Torino* in Turin, Italy
- *University of California* in Davis, CA

According to a study by U.S. governmental Centers for Disease Control and Prevention (CDC), those with a lovely cat or dog on their side tested much less positive for stress and anxiety. Scientifically validated recently at the *University of Florida* in Gainesville.

Writing

Writing down to express what frightens you, e.g. by journaling, makes it easier to cope with anxiety.

Based on research at, inter alia, *Queen's University* in Kingston, Canada.

Aromatherapy

To smell soothing plant oils may well relieve anxiety and stress.

With special reference to lavender. According to research, inter alia, in Taiwan's capital Taipei at
- *Taipei Medical University*
- *National Taipei Medical University of Nursing and Health Sciences*
  &
- *Taipei Medical University Hospital*

IN A NUTSHELL

Anxiety is one of most prevalent and manifold stress-related mental issues in our society. Fortunately, there are natural ways for relief by adjusting our lifestyle accordingly. For self-application, and without sophisticated therapies.

37. CUT DOWN CALORIES – NOT YOUR HEALTH!

THE PHILOSOPHY BEHIND

It has certainly become more or less a kind of golden formula that cutting calories by the numbers is the basic prerequisite for weight control. Unlike manifold understanding, however, dropping calories is by far not necessarily a matter of dietary quantity alone. Rather, the *quality* of food we consume is what really counts. Especially, as we need to make sure that our body (and mind) is well supported and supplied nutritiously. In other words, reducing the amount of calories must not mean to lose the nutritious value of the food we consume. With special reference to vitamins, minerals, dietary fiber, etc.

To make sure which natural foods are healthy in this respect, i.e. nutrient-dense but still low in terms of calories, let us ask the

U.S. DEPARTMENT OF AGRICULTURE

National Nutrient Database as follows. With special reference to more than 3 dozens fruits and vegetables, as follows.

Fruits

- *Apricots*

One raw apricot (weight some 35 grams) is not only rich in vitamins B/C/E/K but still has only 16 calories.

- *Apples*

They are an excellent source of, inter alia, vitamin C & dietary fiber – supporting the health of our gut.

With only 86 calories for small kinds of this fruit.

Similar

- *Grapefruits*

as a nutritiously rich food – expressively in terms of vitamin C - but only 10 calories per slice.

- *Watermelon*

This is a very good source of vitamins A/B-6/C, with 10 balls of watermelon having just 37 calories.

- *Strawberries*

With a rich portfolio of vitamin C, manganese, antioxidants and dietary fiber, one single piece of this fruit has got just 6 calories.

Also

- *Raspberries*

are very nutritious in terms of vitamins C&K, manganese and dietary fiber.

Still, one cup of this fruit (150 grams) has got just 78 calories.

- *Papaya*

100 grams of this fruit not only offer 70% of vitamin C as needed daily by adults, but has got just 43 calories.

- *Cherries*

Rich in vitamins like vitamin C, potassium and fiber, one cup of 150 grams has got only 95 calories.

- *Lychees*

As a rich source of vitamin C, one lychee comes with only 7 calories.

Vegetables

- *Spinach*

is rich in vitamins A/B-6/C and vital minerals (such as iron and manganese) but still has got only 6 calories per cup of 25 grams.

Also

- *Kale*

is rich in vitamins (C&K), along with calcium, iron and fiber, with only 9 calories per 25-g cup.

- *Watercress*

Rich in nutrients such as vitamins A/C/E/K and calcium, one cup of 34 grams chopped watercress has less than 4 calories.

- *Zucchini*

While this well-known vegetable is rich in terms of vitamin C, dietary fiber and potassium, one serving with 95 grams has got only 20 calories.

- *Asparagus*

Powerful in vitamins A/E/K and the vital mineral iron, one spear of this healthy vegetable has only 3 calories, and one cup (with 134 grams) still not more than 27 calories.

- *Tomatoes*

This vegetable is not only high in vitamins C&K, also potassium and folate.

It's got just 25 calories for a serving of 126 grams.

Similar

- *Fennel*

Equally rich in vitamins C&K and potassium, as well as an excellent source of dietary fiber, got only 36 calories per half of a bulb.

- *Iceberg lettuce*

Rich in vitamins A&K, and folate, one cup (72 grams) of shredded lettuce has got only 10 calories.

Also

- *Cucumber*

is powerful in terms of vitamin K, with only 18 calories per shredded cup of 120 grams.

- *Celery*

Rich in antioxidants like vitamin C and flavonoids, one stalk of celery got less than 6 calories.

Mineral-rich

- *Arugula*

(in terms of potassium/calcium/iron) contains no more than t5 calories per cup of 20 grams.

- *Beets*

Just one beet of 80 grams, on the other hand, is rich in vitamin C, folate and dietary fiber, but contains only 34 calories.

- *Alfalfa sprouts*

Rich in B-vitamins & vitamin K, as well as minerals copper and zinc, got only 8 calories per cup of 33 grams.

- *Peppers*

Loaded with vitamins B-6 & C, a service of 85 grams has only 25 calories.

- *Olives*

Green/black olives, one side are rich in vitamin E and minerals of calcium and iron, on the other, however, have only 22 calories in a serving of 15 grams.

- *Cauliflower*

Powerful in vitamin C, one cup (100 grams) of this vegetable comes with 5 grams of carbohydrates and 27 calories.

- *Broccoli*

Besides fiber, this well -known vegetable contains many vitamins (A/B&B-9/C/E/K) and minerals (calcium & magnesium). Still, calories are limited to 30 per cup of 90 grams broccoli florets.

- *Turnip*

Rich in vitamins (B-6&C) and minerals (calcium & potassium), as well as dietary fiber, in one cup of 130 grams there are only 36 calories.

- *Carrots*

Loaded with vitamins (B/C/K), one small carrot with 5.5 inches comes with only 20 calories.

Another rooted vegetable named

- *Rutabaga*

is rich in vitamins (C & E) and minerals (magnesium/calcium/potassium) with only 50 calories per cup of 140 grams.

- *Chard*

This nutrient-dense vegetable, loaded with vitamins (B-6/C/E/K), minerals (iron and calcium) and fiber, has only 19 calories per serving of 100 grams.

Also

- *Leeks*

Contain minerals iron and calcium, along with vitamins B&C, with 55 calories for a standard size.

Although

- *Pumpkin*

is rich in vitamins A//B-6/C/E, a cup with 116 grams has got only 30 calories.

- *Green beans*

Rich in vitamins B/C/K, a cup of 100 grams green beans comes up with 31 calories only.

Similar to

- *Okra*

with 33 calories per 100 grams, but rich in vitamins A & B-9 and magnesium.

- *Onions*

(red and white) known for vitamins B-6 & C, have something between 40 and 45 calories for a serving of 100 grams.

- *Brussels sprouts*

A cup of 100 grams is not only rich in vitamins C & K has got only 39 calories per 100-g cup.

- *Radishes*

As an excellent source of vitamins B-9 & C as well as potassium, they have only 18 calories per 116-gram cup sliced.

- *Red cabbage*

Rich in vitamins A/C/K, 70 grams in shredded form got only 22 calories.

Not to overlook

- *White mushrooms*

As a powerful source of, inter alia, vitamin D and zinc, 35 grams (1/2 cup) in sliced form, they got less than 8 calories.

IN A NUTSHELL

Cutting calories for losing weight may well be a magic formula. Provided, we still get those nutrients vital for our health. Learn about more than 3 dozens of natural foods with high nutritional profile but limited calories.

38. HIGH BLOOD PRESSURE: FOODS TO LIMIT

THE PHILOSOPHY BEHIND

As you have learned from our previous blogs, more than 80% of non-age-related deaths and more than three quarters of all ailments in general, are the consequence of unsolved disease. According to the *World Health Organization (WHO)*. With heart failure on top of the list – caused primarily by high blood pressure. In fact, based on findings of the U.S. *Centers for Disease Control and Prevention (CDC)*, almost half of adults in this country are suffering from hypertension which increases the risk of heart disease and stroke.

While there are different natural remedies and modalities to tackle this vicious cycle, it is equally important to...

LIMIT CERTAIN FOODS – SCIENTIFICALLY VALIDATED

...for better control of high blood pressure. Inter alia...

Sodium-rich foods

According to the *Centers for Disease Control and Prevention (CDC)* we should limit daily sodium consumption with no more than 2,3 milligrams.

Unfortunately, this is highly surpassed in many cases of processed/fast foods like
- sandwiches
- pizzas
- tacos & burritos
- rolls & bread
- canned soup
- cold cuts & cured meats

which may even elevate blood pressure.

Also

Red meat

of different kinds may well increase high blood pressure. Not only
- beef

- pork
- veal
  but also
- venison
- lamb
- goat

Based on research at, inter alia, at the *University of Illinois* in Chicago, IL.

Saturated fats

Although not completely prohibited, in order to lower high blood pressure, the *American Heart Association (AHA)* recommends to consume no more than 6% of calories per day from saturated fats derived from, inter alia,

- desserts
  (chocolate/cakes/biscuits/pies/pastries/cakes/pudding/etc.)
- full-fat dairy products
  (milk/cheese/yogurt/cream/crème fraiche/etc.)
- processed meat
  (burgers/sausages/bacon/kebabs/etc.)
- cooking fats
  (butter/margarine/ghee/lard/goose fat/suet, etc.)
- oils
  (coconut oil/palm oils/etc.)

Sugary drinks

These drinks may intensify high blood pressure. Especially if they contain high fructose corn syrup or caffeine like some sodas and fruit juices.

Caffeine may raise blood pressure considerably at least temporarily.

Based on research at, inter alia,
- *Albert Einstein College of Medicine, Montefiore Medical Center* in Bronx, NY
  &
- *Saint Luke's Mid America Heart Institute* in Kansas City, Missouri

Similar the situation (and partly worse than in cases of sodium-rich foods) with

Sugary foods

according to same research. With special reference to high fructose corn syrup.

Including, inter alia,
- processed/prepackaged meals (like vegetables & meat-based meals)
- peanut butter
- granola & other nutrition bars
- crackers

HOWEVER...

...to *limit* certain nutrition does not mean to abdicate some delicious food.

Rather, to replace it by other delicious – but blood-pressure-friendly – nutrition, as recommended inter alia by the U.S. *National Heart, Lung, and Blood Institute* as an example:
- whole grains
- fruits (like berries/citrus fruits/avocados/etc.)
- vegetables (like leafy greens/etc.)
- fish
- lean meats (like grilled chicken/chicken breast)
- poultry
- protein sources (like nuts/lentils/quinoa/tofu/etc.)

IN A NUTSHELL

According to the *World Health Organization (WHO)*, more than 80% of non-age-related deaths and more than three quarters of all ailments in general, are the consequence of conventionally unsolved disease. With heart failure on top of the list – caused primarily by high blood pressure. To tackle this vicious cycle naturally, limit certain foods, as recommended, scientifically verified.

39. WHICH DIET BETTER FOR YOUR HEALTH?

THE PHILOSOPHY BEHIND

As you have learned not only – but also – from our publications, the central criterion responsible for our health and longevity is our immune system. As the complex power of biologic natural laws in our body. Scientifically validated in the U.S. and internationally. Inter alia, in Canada at

- *University of Manitoba* (Winnipeg, MB)
- *Western University* (London, ON)
- *McMaster University* (Hamilton, ON)
- *Dalhousie University* (Halifax, NS)

With 2 lines of defense: *innate* & *adaptive* immunity.

Thereby, the innate immunity is the *first* line of defense with its physical barriers like the skin, as well as chemical and cellular defenses, making no difference between foreign invaders.

If in this case, the innate immunity is not sufficiently effective, the adaptive immunity gets in charge. With its specific blood cells and proteins to fight the infection. And since it has got a kind of 'memory', it targets the same infection should it happen later again.

This implies that support of our immune system is vital. Provided, we support our immune system naturally. With diet in the forefront. Which diet?

DIET FOR HEALTH – GOOD & BAD – SCIENTIFICALLY VERIFIED

Western diet

Unfortunately, 'Western' diet, as we are overwhelmingly used to it, may still not be the answer. With its highly processed foods and beverages (including sodas), rich in refined carbohydrates and calories, with special reference to saturated fats, and added sugar/salt. Thus inducing inflammation and risk of (manifold chronic) disease.

According to international research at, inter alia, the *University of Bonn* in Bonn, Germany, and *Federico II University Medical School of Naples* in Naples, Italy.

With a negative impact also on our blood sugar, potentially resulting in diabetes, according to international research at
- *Leiden University Medical Center* in Leiden, The Netherlands
- *Post Graduate Institute of Medical Education and Research* in Chandigarh, India
- *Korea Food Research Institute* in Jeollabuk-do, South Korea

This is also raising inflammation proteins, including C-reactive protein (CRP), tumor necrosis-alpha (TNF-alpha) and interleukin-6 (IL-6).

Based on international research at, inter alia,
- *I.M. Sechenov First Moscow Medical University* in Moscow, Russia
- *University of Sao Paulo* in Sao Paulo, Brazil
- *University of Southampton* in Southampton, UK
- *California Polytechnic State University* in San Luis Obispo, California
  &
- *Luxembourg Institute of Health* in Strassen, Luxembourg

Including autoimmune diseases like rheumatoid arthritis, according to research at, inter alia,
- *Universite Paris* in Paris, France
- *Universite de Nice Sophia-Antipolis* in Nice, France

As verified scientifically internationally also at, inter alia, the
- *University of Bonn* in Bonn, Germany
- *University of Massachusetts Medical School* in Worcester, Massachusetts
  &
- *Norwegian University of Science and Technology* in Trondheim, Norway

Mediterranean diet

As indicated above, ultra-processed food high in calories, with special reference to saturated fats and excessively added sugar and salt, do not support our immune system – and health/longevity accordingly.

Other than whole, nutrient-dense foods like fruits, vegetables, legumes, seafood and nuts, with special reference to vitamins C & D and zinc. According to international research at, inter alia, the *Federico II University Medical School of Naples* in Naples, Italy, and *Universidade de Sao Paulo* in Sao Paulo, Brazil.

Based on this background, especially Mediterranean diet (although part of 'Western' hemisphere) has proven highly beneficial by lowering the risk of inflammation and (chronic) disease.

According to international medical research at, inter alia, the
- *University of Barcelona* in Barcelona, Spain –
- *Wake Forest School of Medicine* in Winston-Salem, North Carolina &
- *Oregon State University* in Corvallis, Oregon

With special reference to vital nutrients such as vitamins A/B-6/B-9/B-12/C/D as well as zinc, selenium, iron and high dietary fiber. Richly found in Mediterranean diet. Reducing the risk of infections.

Again, according to research at, inter alia, *Oregon State University* in Corvallis, Oregon.

Not only this. Mediterranean diet with special reference to fruits and vegetables are cutting down markers of chronic inflammation as IL-6, CRP and fibrinogen and strengthening the immune system, accordingly.

Based on research at, inter alia, *Wageningen University and Research* in Wageningen, The Netherlands.

Rounding up with healthy lifestyle including, inter alia,
- physical activity
- restful sleep &
- stress reduction

IN A NUTSHELL

Our health and longevity depends on a strong and powerful immune system warding off infections. For best support, besides certain lifestyle factors, healthy diet plays a decisive role. With nutrients we better don't miss. As basically indicated in this chapter. Scientifically validated.

40. BETA-BLOCKERS FOR HEART: ASK NATURE

THE PHILOSOPHY BEHIND

According to the *World Health Organization (WHO)* & validated also by the U.S. *Centers for Disease Control and Prevention (CDC)*, more than 80% of non-age-related premature deaths are the consequence of unsolved health issues. With heart failure leading this vicious cycle (followed by cancer).

Based on this background, usually synthetic beta-blockers are prescribed, to block certain hormones in the nervous system responsible for stress on the heart. In order to reduce high blood pressure and other cardiovascular health issues. Related to manifold debilitating side effects.

NATURAL ALTERNATIVES – SCIENTIFICALLY VALIDATED

Fortunately, nature got alternatives to replace these synthetics – no less powerful and without debilitating side effects. According to research at, inter alia, the *University of Iowa Hospitals and Clinics* in Iowa City, IA, and *Drexel University* in Philadelphia, PA.

With special reference to high blood pressure – and other cardiovascular health issues such as, inter alia:
- stroke
- irregular heartbeat (arrhythmia)
- resting heartbeat (tachycardia)
- congestive heart failure
- coronary artery disease
- aortic dissection (tearing in aorta lining)

And additionally, based on this research, these natural blockers may even help with
- anxiety
- migraine
- glaucoma
- certain tremors
- portal hypertension

Just let's pick some of those natural beta-blockers – scientifically validated:

Celery

With special reference to the compounds of apigenin and n-butylphthalide, this familiar vegetable, reducing adrenaline and noradrenaline, cuts down force of pumping blood throughout the body and blood pressure, accordingly. Thus reducing stress on the heart.

Garlic

Based on heart-healthy constituents like manganese, selenium, and vitamins B-6 & C, and the antioxidant allicin, according to the *British Heart Foundation,* it controls blood pressure as well. Scientifically verified, inter alia, in Australia at
- *Torrens University* in Melbourne
- *University of Adelaide* in Adelaide
  and the
- *National Institute of Integrative Medicine* in Melbourne

Similar the situation with

Pulses

such as beans, chickpeas and lentils. As their protein, fiber and potassium helps lowering high blood pressure.

According to research at, inter alia,
- *Pennsylvania State University* in University Park, PA
- *Harvard School of Public Health* in Boston, MA
- *Cleveland Clinic* in Lyndhurst, OH
  as well as following Canadian institutions:
- *University of Saskatchewan* in Saskatoon,
- *McMaster University* in Hamilton,
- *University of Toronto* in Toronto
- *St. Michael's Hospital* in Toronto
- *Heart and Stroke Foundation of Ontario* in Toronto

With respect to fruit as a natural source of beta-blockers, the U.S. *National Institutes of Health (NIH)* recommends

Hawthorn berries

not only as a natural beta-blocker but also as a calcium-channel-blocker, diuretic, and angiotensin-converting enzyme inhibitor.

Hibiscus

This herb is not only known in folk medicine to cut down high blood pressure but has been scientifically verified in this capacity at, inter alia, the *American University of Beirut* in Beirut, Lebanon and *Qatar University* in Doha, Qatar.

According to same scientific reference, also the spice

Saffron

is lowering blood pressure by relaxing/dilating blood vessels.

Vitamin B-6

as we find it, inter alia, in starchy vegetables, most fruits, poultry and fish, etc., is widening blood vessels in favor of our blood pressure.

According to the U.S. *National Institutes of Health (NIH)*.

This U.S. governmental source also recommends

Potassium

as an excellent natural blocker as we find it, inter alia, in foods like
- bananas
- low fat dairy
- coconut water
  and
- potatoes

is widening blood vessels as well as lowering blood pressure, accordingly.

L-arginine

This semi-essential amino acid can be found, inter alia, in different natural foods like, leafy green vegetables, poultry, nuts, and seeds.

According to research at, inter alia, the *National University of Health Sciences* in Lombard, IL, it can reduce both – systolic & diastolic – blood pressure in adults.

Not to forget about

Omega-3 fatty acids

especially found richly in fish like salmon, trout, and herring, as they are reducing the risk of heart disease in general.

According to the *American Heart Association (AHA)*.

IN A NUTSHELL

Based on the fact that cardiovascular diseases are prime in our modern civilized society, manifold synthetic beta-blockers are prescribed. With debilitating side effects. Fortunately, nature offers us many equally powerful alternatives. Any risks and side effects involved with these natural beta-blockers? If consumed in a moderate way and if no allergies are involved, no risks and/or side effects are known. As demonstrated in this blog, scientifically validated.

41. SUPPORT YOUR HEALTH WITH WINE?

THE PHILOSOPHY BEHIND

As you have learned from our previous publications, fruits are basically part of healthy nutrition. Grapes being no exception, with fermentation as a wine included, if consumed in moderation. I.e. up to 2 drinks per day for males and one drink for females, according to the U.S. *Centers for Disease Control and Prevention (CDC)*. Although different types of wines may offer different benefits. And some risks by increasing calories and especially with excessive intake of alcohol.

Basically, the benefits for health come with the content of antioxidants like *polyphenols* in grape skin, preventing damage of cells and inflammation.

As scientifically validated by, inter alia, the
- *University of Houston*
- *Methodist Neurological Institute and Research Institute*
  &
- *Methodist Hospital*
  (all in Houston, Texas)
  as well as
- *Cornell University* in New York, NY
  &
- *University of Strasbourg* in Strasbourg, France

Not enough. With special reference to the fact that most polyphenols are flavonoids, wine has been identified to also help in cases of cancer by slowing tumor cell growth, and inhibit absorption of glucose in cases of diabetes.

Based on research at, inter alia, *Universidade do Porto* in Porto, Portugal.

However, these benefits have to be seen in relation to moderate wine consumption. Otherwise, i.e. with excessive consumption, this may potentially lead to health issues such as, inter alia, liver damage, cancer and problems for the fetus during pregnancy.

According to the governmental U.S. *Centers for Disease Control and Prevention (CDC)*.

PROS & CONS OF WINES – SCIENTIFICALLY VALIDATED

Since 7 billion inhabitants on this globe, the Earth, have 7 billion different/individual metabolisms, that's why any benefits and risks involved are always 'potential'.

Thereby, these potential pros and cons of wine depend on the specific type ('color') of grapes, to focus on red and white wine briefly in following. Based on international research.

Red wine

Independent of all kinds of red wine well known worldwide.

Benefits

- ***Heart health***

According to the *American Heart Association (AHA)*, the moderate consumption of red wine may well reduce the risk of mortality in cases of heart disease.

This is especially true because of the antioxidant named *resveratrol* in the skin of red grapes activated during the fermentation process.

With special reference to resveratrol's capacity of
- anti-inflammatory activity
- anti-oxidant activity
- protection against neurodegenerative conditions
- anticancer activity

According to research at, inter alia, the *Lithunian University of Health Sciences* in Kaunas, Lithunia.

More than that. Based on research at, inter alia, the *University College London,* UK, already one glass of red wine daily can support healthy aging with lowering the risk not only of diabetes 2, obesity, cancer, and neurodegenerative diseases but also of cardiovascular disease.

Based on research at the *University of Naples* in Naples, Italy, red wine may also help avoiding atherosclerosis and high blood pressure (hypertension). Scientifically validated, inter alia, by the *Commonwealth Scientific and Industrial Research Organisation* in Adelaide, Australia.

With reference to the benefit of improving heart rhythms and avoiding blood clotting with grapes and their phenol resveratrol to prevent

cardiovascular diseases. Scientifically verified by *Michigan State University* in East Lansing and the *University of Michigan* in Ann Arbor, MI.

This may also explain the philosophy behind *United Nations Development Program (UNDP)* statistics in terms of life expectancy. With wine favoring Mediterranean countries like France, Italy and Spain ranking in top dozen, while the U.S. is lagging behind at position 38.

- **Multiple sclerosis**

According to research at, inter alia,
- *Harvard Medical School*
  &
- *Brigham and Women's Hospital*
  as well as the
- *Multiple Sclerosis Center* at *Massachusetts General Hospital*
  all in Boston, MA

the consumption of red wine may reduce disability of patients struck with multiple sclerosis.

Another benefit of red wine's flavonoids is for the neurodegenerative condition of

- **Alzheimer's disease**

by inhibiting the formation of proteins responsible for this disease.

Based on research at, inter alia, *Clark University* in Worcester, MA.

- **Gut health**

Red wine may also support regulating gut bacteria. According to research in Australia, at the *University of Canberra* and the *University of Melbourne.*

Not to overlook finally that red wine's flavonoids may well protect against

- **Diabetes 2**

According to research at, inter alia, in Boston, MA, at
- *Harvard T.H. Chan School of Public Health*

- *Brigham and Women's Hospital*
- *Harvard Medical School*

- *Massachusetts General Hospital*
  as well as
- *Hospital del Mar Medical Research Institute* in Barcelona
  &
- *Virgili University* in Reus
  (both Spain)

Risks

According to the governmental *Centers of Disease Control and Prevention (CDC)*, in the U.S. alone, there are almost 100,000 mortalities per year due to alcohol intake in large amounts.

Potentially leading to, inter alia, not only

- Short-term to
  - alcohol poisoning
  - injuries
  - miscarriage
  - violence

but also to

- Long-term implications such as
  - heart disease
  - high blood pressure
  - cancer
  - mental health problems
  - weakening of the immune system
  - liver disease
  - alcohol use disorder

White wine

Again, independent of its specific types.

Benefits

Although there is less research on the health benefits of polyphenols in white wine as it is on red, there are at least 2 benefits we don't want to overlook.

- ***Alzheimer's disease***

I.e., that also polyphenols in white wine seem to reduce chronic inflammation in cases of Alzheimer's disease.

According to research in Portugal at the
- *University of Coimbra* in Coimbra
- *Universidade de Porto* in Porto
  &
- *University of Tras-os-Montes e Alto Douro* in Vila Real

- ***Kidney health***

Based on the polyphenol *caffeic acid,* as to be found in white wine, supports the release of nitric oxide from endothelial cells in favor of kidney health.

According to comprehensive research in Italy at, inter alia,
- *University of Milan*
- *University of Pisa*
- *University of Torino*
  &
- *Versilia Hospital* in Lido di Camaiore

Risks

Especially with reference to skin conditions, when consuming white wine with larger amounts of alcohol.

Inter alia,

- ***Melanoma***

as a kind of skin cancer, according to research at
- *Harvard Medical School*
  &
- *Brigham and Women's Hospital*
  both in Boston, MA

- ***Acne***

is another type of skin issue (known by the medical term of *rosacea*) potentially caused by higher amounts of alcohol in white wine in women.

According to research at, inter alia,
- *Harvard Medical School*
  &
- *Brigham and Women's Hospital*
  both in Boston, MA
  as well as
- *Brown University* in Providence, RI
  &
- *Shandong University* in Jinan, China

Not to overlook

- **Weight gain**

in cases of excessive white wine consumption with potentially high calorie intake, respectively.

Based on the benchmark that, according to the *Agricultural Research Service* of the *U.S. Department of Agriculture (USDA),* one glass of white wine comes usually with 148 calories.

IN A NUTSHELL

Like fruits in general, the moderate consumption also of fermented grapes in form of wine, is basically beneficial for our health. Although rounded up with some risks in cases of (excessive) alcohol intake. As demonstrated in this chapter with reference to red and white wine, scientifically verified.

42. PROS & CONS OF FRUITS FOR YOUR HEALTH

THE PHILOSOPHY BEHIND

To stay healthy during long life, our diet containing whole foods with vital nutrients is of central importance. With special reference to plants as vegetables and fruits. That's why, e.g., the Mediterranean diet, including lots of whole foods such as fruits, vegetables and whole grain, is of basic relevance for health and longevity.

Period? Almost. Because 7 billion inhabitants of this planet, the Earth, have got 7 billion individual metabolisms. This implies that we do not only need nutrients for our health but this needs to be in line with our individual status of health.

However, not all fruits are of same relevance in cases of certain health conditions in general. I.e., some fruits may be more important than others or may be better to avoid in certain individual cases of individual health conditions, allergies, or lifestyle factors.

E.g., some fruits are basically high in dietary sugar, raising blood sugar, with reference to the fact that these fruits are problematic for diabetics. Other fruits are rich in fats with respect to higher calory level, being crucial for weight loss, etc.

Therefore, it is important to understand individually, if certain health-related disadvantages overweigh the benefits of certain fruits.

VALIDATED BENEFITS AND LIMITS BY USDA-FNDDS

Let's focus on pros and cons of following sample of certain fruits with reference to the *U.S. Department of Agriculture's Food and Nutrient Database (FNDDS)*. To understand not only their overall benefits but also potential disadvantages for your health individually.

Bananas

On one side, bananas are rich of very important nutrients, especially

- vitamins B-6 & C
  as well as
- minerals

- potassium
- magnesium
- copper

But on the other, they contain amounts of
- sugar
- carbs
- fats
- calories

which are less favorable in cases of specific health issues like, e.g., diabetes.

Although bananas do have also fiber – but not richly enough to counterbalance the sugar.

Like

Grapes

They contain vitamin C as well as calcium and copper, but not enough fiber for making good the sugar content.

Similar the situation with

Mangoes

as they are not only rich in

- vitamins A/B-6/C
  &
- minerals potassium & copper

but also come with high levels of sugar and therefore, less favorable for diabetics as well. Despite of containing some fiber, but – again – not enough to balance out the sugar.

Same with

Lychees

As a good source of vitamin C as well as minerals potassium and copper, their fiber is still not high enough to balance out the sugar content as well.

Cherries

are containing
- vitamin C
&
- minerals calcium & iron

but, unfortunately, are rich in sugar as well and therefore not an optimal choice for diabetics.

Coconuts

Although coconuts are an excellent source of minerals such as
- magnesium
- potassium
- calcium
- iron
&
- selenium

plus vitamin C, they are not the #1 choice to reduce fat and calories.

Any well-balanced alternatives?

How's about ...

Berries

These fruits are not only high of antioxidants beneficial for overall health. Berries are traditionally low in sugar on one side, on the other they are rich in vitamins and fiber.

Based on this background, they help with weight loss, lower the level of calories and, according to a recent meta-analysis published in the medical journal *Nutrients*, it's cutting the risk of cardiovascular disease, diabetes, metabolic syndrome, and cancer.

Watermelons

Rich in vitamins A & C, as well as potassium, they are also sweet without any disadvantage for diabetics, and without any other known health issue.

Also beneficial for our health in general is the

Grapefruit

This fruit is low in calories but rich in
- vitamins A&C

as well as
-    minerals calcium, potassium & magnesium
as an all-rounder fruit for our health.

Not to forget about the 'king of the road':

Apples

This fruit is an excellent source of antioxidants, with special reference to vitamins such as beta-carotene (as a precursor of vitamin A) and vitamin C, as well as minerals calcium, magnesium and potassium, and fiber.

That's where the philosophy behind of one highly renowned American saying is coming from:

"An apple a day keeps the doctor away."

IN A NUTSHELL

Fruits should be part of our healthy diet. Because of many vital nutrients involved, like vitamins and minerals. However, since 7 billion inhabitants of our planet - the Earth - have 7 billion different (individual) metabolisms, it is also important to balance the respective dietary fruit intake with individual potential health issues involved. With special reference to, inter alia, sugar, fats and calories. In this blog you learn about pros and cons of some fruits regarding this potentially problematic relationship.

43. SUPPORT YOUR IMMUNE SYSTEM WITH DIET?

THE PHILOSOPHY BEHIND

As you have learned from some of our previous publications, health and longevity are basically dependent on a strong immune system – and how to support this prerequisite. Needless to stress that our daily nutrition plays a decisive role in this context. In both directions. I.e., there are foods highly supportive for our immune system, and others which are not. To find our right way through this discrepancy, we shall focus on some differences between healthy and unhealthy food for our immune system in following. Basically a kind of blueprint between *Western* & Mediterran*ean* diet. As scientifically verified, inter alia, at the *University Center for the Defense of Madrid* in Spain's capital Madrid.

IMMUNITY SUPPORTING FOODS

- ### *Cruciferous vegetables*

Based on the substance *sulphoraphane,* this vegetable – especially in form of broccoli – is boosting the immune system with anti-inflammatory and even anti-*cancer* power (colon cancer included).

According to international research at *Tel-Aviv University* in Ramat Aviv, Israel, verified by the U.S. *National Institutes of Health* in Bethesda, MD.

- ### *Ginger*

Well known as a spice for dietary flavor since centuries, now medical science identified its power for strengthening also our immune system.

With special reference to fighting inflammation in, inter alia, *osteoarthritis* and *rheumatoid arthritis.*

Based on international research at, inter alia, *Seoul National University* in Seoul, South Korea, and *Vietnam National University* in Ho Chi Minh City, Vietnam.

Not to overlook foods containing

- ### *Zinc*

like, inter alia,
- baked beans
- fortified cereals
- oysters
- peas
- cheese
- beef
- chicken breast

as this essential mineral is most important to support our immune system.

According to research at, inter alia, the *RWTH University* in Aachen, Germany, and verified by the U.S. *National Institutes of Health (NIH)*.

- ***Citrus fruits***

Based on its high content of vitamin C, citrus fruits have been scientifically verified to support our immune system, preferably with a daily consumption of 100-200 mg of vitamin C.

Based on research at, inter alia, the *University of Otago* in Christchurch, New Zealand.

IMMUNITY IMPAIRING FOODS

On the other hand, there are indeed foods we should limit or even avoid when it comes to our immune system. According to the U.S. *National Institutes of Health (NIH)*.

With special reference to

- ***Processed foods***

which contain manifold sugars, unhealthy fats, and additives in
- canned foods
- cakes and cookies
- microwaveable meals
  and/or
- chips

In fact, foods with additives are highly risky for *chronic inflammation, obesity* and *insulin resistance*.

According to international research at, inter alia, *Universidade Federal do Rio de Janeiro* in Rio de Janeiro, Brazil.

Especially, if a shortage of omega-3 fatty acids is involved at the same time. As verified by the U.S. *National Institutes of Health (NIH)*.

Not enough. This type of unhealthy food can also lead to increased consumption of calories with the result of obesity. Potentially causing *inflammation* with insulin resistance and *dysregulation of the immune system*.

Based on research at *Shiraz University of Medical Sciences* in Shiraz, Iran, and the *University of Kiel* in Kiel, Germany.

If processed foods also have high content of refined carbohydrates like, inter alia,
- white bread
- white rice
  and/or
- cookies/cakes/sweets

produced with white flour & refined sugar, this can lead to *inflammation* and *oxidative stress*, harming the immune system.

According to international research at, inter alia,
- *California Polytechnic State University* in San Luis Obispo, CA
- *I.M. Sechenov First Moscow Medical University* in Russia's capital Moscow
  &
- *Luxembourg Institute of Health* in Strassen, Luxembourg.

- ***Foods with high sugar content***

High sugar intake increases the risk of, inter alia, *diabetes 2* and *coronary heart disease*.

According to international research at, inter alia,
- *Saint Luke's Mid America Heart Institute* in Kansas City, MO
- *Albert Einstein College of Medicine / Montefiori Medical Center* in Bronx, NY
  &
- *Ospedale Generale* in Bolzano, Italy

With special reference to following foods:
- flavored milk
- sweetened dairy products

-    sugary breakfast cereals
-    cookies/cakes
-    preserves/marmalades/sweets
  &
-    sugary drinks

Even more. According to the *American Cancer Society*, sugary drinks may double the risk of bowel cancer in cases of women aged under 50.

IN A NUTSHELL

To support health and longevity, our immune system is the central force to accomplish. Doing justice accordingly, certain foods are of high importance, just as others turn out counterproductive. To understand this discrepancy, we are focusing on a sample of basic pros and cons. All scientifically verified.

44. RELIEVE ARTHRITIS WITH NATURE

THE PHILOSOPHY BEHIND

The U.S. is foremost in conventional medicine, spending most for medicine per capita. Still, 86% of non-age-related deaths and 77% of ailments in general are the consequence of *chronic* - speak: unsolved - diseases.

One of those health issues is arthritis with some 100 different types. More than 50 million Americans being affected. With special reference to

- osteoarthritis (OA) - when the cartilage of joints are wearing out, leading to a change of bones. Causing swelling, stiffness – and pain.
  &
- rheumatoid arthritis (RA) as an inflammatory disease, when the immune system attacks healthy tissues, affecting also several joints at same time even on both sides of the body.

NATURAL TREATMENTS – SCIENTIFICALLY VERIFIED

While conventional medicine has not found a solution yet, nature offers us well some therapies to relieve swelling, stiffness – and pain. With special reference to certain lifestyle and dietary adjustments – at no or almost no cost. In many cases to be applied at your own home.

Just to cover briefly half a dozen of those lifestyle & dietary therapies out of nature's comprehensive portfolio in following.

Physical therapy

With special reference to rheumatoid arthritis, *Inje University* at the Republic of Korea, came to positive conclusions in their research.

As far as, primarily,
- range of motion like getting in and out of chairs, climbing stairs, walking in your neighborhood, playing a sport or doing recreational activities,
  but also
- rebuilding strength
- correct posture
- improvement of coordination

and above all
- pain relief

is concerned.

Especially, as this natural physical therapy came to better results than standard rheumatology.

- Swimming

This type of physical movement eases the joints as it relieves the effect of gravity on the movements of the body. Accordingly, swimming does gently move the respective joints, keeping muscles strong.

In fact, this impact on endurance, strength, balance, and stretching relieves pain.

According to research at, inter alia, the *University of Utah* in Salt Lake City, Utah.

Weight loss

Some 80% of Americans struck with arthritis are overweight or obese, according to the U.S. *Centers for Disease Control and Prevention (CDC).*

Not only is pressure on joints one-and-a-half times the personal body weight, with each step on flat surface. In case of arthritis the pressure on joints is raised up to 4 times the body weight. Based on findings of the U.S. *Arthritis Foundation.*

The good news is that, with any loss of 5 pound body weight, the stress on joints is reduced by 20% - with a significant pain relief as a result.

Therefore, lose weight, accordingly especially in cases of arthritis.

Massage

According to the U.S. *National Center for Complementary and Integrative Health (NIH),* one hour of whole-body massage may well improve symptoms of knee osteoarthritis even on a short-term basis, with special reference to pain and stiffness. Improving joint function as well.

Mindfulness meditation

Based on research at, inter alia, the *University of Auckland* in Auckland, New Zealand, with special reference to rheumatoid arthritis (RA) mindful meditation may relieve pain resulting from chronic symptoms – arthritis included.

Not to overlook

Omega-3 fatty acids

These essential fatty acids are anti-inflammatory.

To be found in healthy diet like, inter alia,
- flax seeds
- chia seeds
- pumpkin seeds
- olive oil
- Brussels sprouts
- soybeans
- spinach
- papaya
- pecans
- walnuts
- eggs
- cod liver oil
- mackerel
- salmon
- sardines

With special reference to rheumatoid arthritis (RA), based on research in Greece at *Asclepeion Hospital* in Athens & *St. Paul's Hospital* in Thessaloniki.

IN A NUTSHELL

While synthetic medicine has not found a satisfactory solution for arthritis yet, nature is offering us quite a few encouraging therapies to relieve arthritis-related swelling, stiffness – and pain. In this chapter you have learned about a sample of these natural therapies based on lifestyle and dietary adjustments. Scientifically verified.

45. DOES CYCLING SUPPORT YOUR HEALTH?

THE PHILOSOPHY BEHIND

As you know from our previous publications, our health and longevity depends primarily on healthy diet and (preferably aerobic) physical exercise. To support our existence in both directions - physically and mentally. Doing justice with respect to physical exercise, there are quite a few opportunities. With riding a bike being one of those. By raising the fitness level at the same time more than with other physical activities. According to international research at, inter alia, the *University of Glasgow* in Glasgow, UK.

With cycling being incorporated easily and economically in daily life. Indoor and outdoor. According to U.S. *Centers for Disease Control and Prevention (CDC).*

HEALTH BENEFITS OF CYCLING – SCIENTIFICALLY VALIDATED

Based on U.S. Federal *Physical Activity Guidelines Advisory Committee,* as verified by the *World Health Organization (WHO),* adults should ride a bike moderately 150-300 minutes or vigorously 75-150 minutes per week. Supported by research at, inter alia, *Harvard Medical School* in Boston, MA.

With following benefits – just to pick 5 out of nature's portfolio...

Cardiovascular health

According to international research at the *University of Glasgow* in Glasgow, UK, regular cycling as recommended above, may cut the risk of cardiovascular disease and dying of it prematurely in half.

In this context, riding the bike regularly may also cut high blood pressure (as one of the causes behind cardiovascular disease) at least over some time. Especially in diabetics.

Based on international research at, inter alia,
- *Einstein Medical Center* in Philadelphia, PA
&
- *Delhi Diabetes Education and Research Foundation* in New Delhi, India

Mental health

As pointed out above, physical exercise is not at all limited to our body but extended to our mental performance at the same time.

Accordingly, all physical exercises have a positive impact on our mental condition as well. Cycling being no exception. With special reference to our cognitive function.

Scientifically verified, inter alia, by research in the UK at
- *University of Reading* in Reading
- *University College London* in London
  &
- *Oxford Brookes University* in Oxford

More than that, according to U.S. Federal *Physical Activity Guidelines Advisory Committee,* cycling may even reduce anxiety and depression.

Lung health

To cycle for 170-250 minutes per week may also support the efficiency of our lung (with & without lung conditions), according to research at, inter alia,
- *Mayo Clinic* in Rochester, Minnesota,
  as well as the
- *Federal University of Fronteira Sul* in Chapeco
  &
- *University of Oeste Paulista (UNOESTE)* in Presidente Prudente
  (both Brazil)

Internationally verified also by the
- *European Lung Foundation* in Sheffield, UK
  &
- *European Respiratory Society* in Lausanne, Switzerland
with special reference to chronic obstructive pulmonary disease (COPD).

Not to forget about

Weight management

since cycling may well reduce our body's mass and fat. In fact, cycling may cut up to 300 calories per hour – and even more by increasing cycling intensity.

According to international research, inter alia in Spain at the

- *Catholic University of Murcia* in Murcia
  &
- *University of Extremadura* in Caceres

IN A NUTSHELL

Our health and longevity depends primarily on healthy diet and physical exercise. Cycling being a supreme choice of physical activities in-and/or outdoor. Resulting in quite a few physical and mental benefits we may not want to miss. Scientifically verified.

46. MONK FRUIT FOR YOUR HEALTH?

THE PHILOSOPHY BEHIND

As you have learned also from our publications and seminars, our health & longevity depends thoroughly on healthy diet. With many different fruits and vegetables in the forefront. Independent of their nativity and heritage on our globe, the Earth. Depending on their content of certain nutrients.

Monk fruit – an inconspicuous looking small round fruit from southern China (named *Luo Hand Guo* there) - being one of those fruits of high quality for our body and mind?

Historic background

This monk fruit is short in calories and carbohydrates, but is a powerful natural sweetener, 300 times stronger than contemporary sugar. Used and cultivated historically by Buddhist Luohan monks already in the 13th century (that's where the name *monk fruit* is derived). Accordingly, it has become part of the Traditional Chinese Medicine (TCM).

HEALTH BENEFITS - SCIENTIFIC VERIFICATION

Monk Fruit helps with lung disease, respiratory problems, sore throats, digestive problems - and

Diabetes

With special reference to this fruit's content of *mogrosides* responsible for its high sweetening power.

Based on comprehensive Chinese research at, inter alia,
- *Peking University*
  &
- *Beijing University of Chinese Medicine*
  (both in China's capital Beijing)
  As well as
- *Municipal People's Hospital* in Hezhou

Confirming that monk fruit is not only is not only powerful to control blood sugar, but is also safe for diabetics.

Not enough. Monk fruit may also have

Anticancer properties

by potentially suppressing growth of throat and colorectal cancers.

As mogrosides with their the antioxidant effect are reducing the DNA damage of free radicals.

According to Chinese research at, inter alia,
- *Beihang University*
  &
- *Beijing University of Agriculture*
  (both in China's capital Beijing)
  as well as
- *Chinese Academy of Sciences* in Tianjin

Anti-inflammatory properties

The fact that mogrosides are protecting from damage by free radicals is *anti-inflammatory,* supporting our body's self-healing power.

This is especially important as *chronic inflammation* is causing many health issues such as, inter alia, heart disease, cancer, diabetes, ulcerative colitis, and Crohn's disease (as a digestive disorder).

Based on research at, inter alia, *Pondicherry University* in Pondicherry, India.

Another potential health benefit of monk fruit may be

Fighting infections

Based on research at, inter alia, the *University of Kentucky* in Lexington, KY.

According to same research results, monk fruit may also fight *candida,* causing painful oral thrush.

Monk fruit is especially powerful in cases when certain germs are resisting the overuse of conventional antibiotics. As verified by the U.S. *Centers for Disease Control and Prevention (CDC).*

Not to overlook that monk fruit can well promote

Weight loss

as it is short of calories and carbohydrates – but an excellent natural sweetener and still very nutritious.

IN A NUTSHELL

Monk fruit – designation derived from the Chinese Buddhist Luohan monks already in the 13th century – is not only free of calories and carbohydrates but an excellent natural sweetener. More than that, this fruit is highly nutritious we would not like to overlook for our health & longevity. Scientifically validated.

47. WHICH DIET IS RAISING RISK OF CANCER?

THE PHILOSOPHY BEHIND

Half a century ago (1971) U.S. President Nixon declared the *War on Cancer*. Still – 86% of non-age-related deaths and 77% of all ailments in general are the consequence of 'chronic' (unsolved) diseases, with cancer topping #2, just behind heart failure. According to the global statistics of the *World Health Organization (WHO)*, and on its way to #1, according to the *International Agency for Research on Cancer (IARC)* in Lyon, France (as part of the *World Health Organization)*.

While causes behind cancer's incidence are manifold, with special reference to environmental problems, **diet** plays a decisive role in this context as well. Not only according to the *National Cancer Institute* of the U.S. *National Institutes of Health* in Bethesda, MD. But also based on international research at, inter alia, the

- *University of Oxford* in Oxford, UK
- *University of Auckland* in Auckland, New Zealand
- *Imperial College London* in London, UK
- *University of Ioannina* in Ioannina, Greece
- *National Cancer Center* in Tokyo, Japan

FOODS INCREASING CANCER RISK – SCIENTIFICALLY VERIFIED

Ultra-processed foods

The problem behind this type of food in relation to cancer's incidence are ingredients like

- high-fructose corn syrup
- artificial sweeteners
- thickeners
- flavor enhancers

resulting from the industrial processing of certain foods (and beverages) – especially those of so called *Western* diet - like

- Breakfast cereals
- Ultra-processed savory and sweet snack foods
- Candy
- Frozen pizzas
- Soda/energy drinks

which are abundant in added sugar and salt, but insufficient in protective nutrients like vitamins, minerals and fiber.

Not only this. In these ultra-processed foods we also find carcinogenic compounds as a result of processing procedure and packaging.

Based on international research at, inter alia
- *Paris 13 University* in Bobigny, France
  &
- *University of Sao Paulo* in Sao Paulo, Brazil

In numbers: based on aforementioned research, ultra-processed food may well enhance risk of cancer by more than 10%.

In this context, let's focus also on

- Red processed meats

as being carcinogenic in particular. With special reference to
- colorectal cancer
- stomach cancer
  &
- breast cancer

According to the *International Agency for Research on Cancer (IARC)* in Lyon, France (as part of the *World Health Organization*).

Scientifically verified, inter alia, at
- *Harvard T.H. Chan School of Public Health* in Boston, MA
  As well as in South Korea at
- *Seoul National University* in Seoul
- *Kangwon National University* in Gangwon-do
  &
- *Dongguk University* in Goyang

Not to overlook also

High-salt- diets

with special reference to stomach and esophageal cancer, as these high-salt-diets may enhance infection.

Based on research at, inter alia,
- *Brown University*
  &

- *Rhode Island Hospital*
  both in Providence, RI

Scientifically verified also by the *International Agency for Research on Cancer (IARC)* in Lyon, France.

Scalding beverages

may not be forgotten to be cancerous as well. Also verified by the *International Agency for Research on Cancer (IARC)* in Lyon, France.

With special reference to hot beverages with temperatures over 149 F/65 C.

According to research at *Huazhong University of Science and Technology* in Wuhan, China.

IN A NUTSHELL

While some environmental impacts are well a cause behind cancer, we may not want to overlook some equally important dietary factors leading to the same negative result. Scientifically verified.

48. HOW PRESS AWAY HEADACHE NATURALLY?

THE PHILOSOPHY BEHIND

Appreciating the fact that our body is a complex biologic-ecologic phenomenon, headache is one of most common symptoms related to health issues generally. Like, inter alia, …
-     stress
-     pain/tension in muscles
-     dehydration
-     allergies
-     fatigue

…just to name a couple of those.

Usually tackled with drugs – leading to additional symptoms and health issues – yes, an unsolved vicious cycle.

To circumvent, *Traditional Chinese Medicine (TCM)* is offering us a natural therapy named *acupressure* to touch certain points on our body softly and powerful, in order to balance the energy system of our body. Alleviating pain – headache included. (Without synthetic drugs.)

TCM PRESSURE POINTS – SCIENTIFICALLY VALIDATED

Although these TCM findings go back thousands of years, they are scientifically verified today. Inter alia in China, by the
-     *University of Science and Technology* in Wuhan
-     *Guangzhou University of Chinese Medicine* in Guangzhou

as well as
-     *I-Shou University*
      &
-     *Kaohsiung Medical University*
      (both in Kaohsiung, Taiwan)

Thereby, to stimulate pressure points, pressure should be firm for several minutes in a circular or up-and-down motion. Without hurting, to be sure.

Let's consider following half dozen pressure points (Chinese terms) – on feet and other parts of the body.

Points on feet

Just focus on 2:

- *Zu Lin Qi*

By practitioners of acupressure, this spot is also termed *Gall Bladder 41.*

This pressure point is located between fourth toe and the pinky toe to move down to the area between knuckles connecting toes to feet.

When stimulating for some minutes with applying pressure to this point, this may help with headaches.

- *Tai Chong*

Here comes the spot called *Liver 3* by acupressure practitioners, on top of the foot. To be found on the webbing between the second and the big toes.

Moving down until hand is level with knuckle. Again, stimulating for some minutes to relax headache and tension. Besides also stress and low back pain.

Additional points

There are 4 other pressure points of relevance to relieve headache naturally. Like...

- *Jian Jing*

A spot named *Gall Bladder 21* by practitioners of acupressure.

By stimulating this point in the middle between neck and shoulders.

Helping not only with neck pain and neck stiffness but also headache. Although not recommended in cases of pregnancy.

- *Feng Chi*

Also termed as *Gall Bladder 20,* to stimulate this pressure point on both sides of the spine, at the spot where the large muscles of the neck attach to the base of the head.

- *Zhong Zu*

Termed *Triple Heater 3* by acupressure practitioners, this spot is between ring and pinky finger, and the knuckles to connect fingers to the hand.

Besides relieving shoulder and neck pain, so it does with tension headaches.

Finally

- *He Gu*

also termed as *Large Intestine 4* to be located at the side of the index finger connecting to the hand, between the index finger and thumb.

This may not only relieve tension, stress, and toothache, but also headaches.

However, it is not safe during pregnancy either.

IN A NUTSHELL

While headache is a common health issue in our times, its relieve the natural way (i.e. without drug-related symptoms and additional health issues) is very uncommon. But Traditional Chinese Medicine (TCM) offers us an easy self-applicable natural therapy.

49. POMELO – WONDER FRUIT FOR HEALTH?

THE PHILOSOPHY BEHIND

Our existence on this globe, the Earth, is a direct function of nature and her laws. With special reference to natural diet of different kind. Including vitamins, minerals, antioxidants and many other nutrients. In all parts and cultures of this world. To just pick one, take a specific type of citrus fruits: *pomelo*. (Scientific term: *C. grandis* or *C.* maxima) Native to South & Southeast Asia – primarily in countries like China, Thailand, Malaysia, and Fiji. Growing up to the size of a cantaloupe.

In fact, *pomelo* is similar to another fruit most of us know or at least have heard about - grapefruit. Just sweeter and less juicy, and in green color. Still, appropriate for man's existence worldwide.

HEALTH BENEFITS OF POMELO – SCIENTIFICALLY VERIFIED

Especially, as we can acquire pomelo also in our culture - at least online and partly grown also in southern U.S. – we should know about its health benefits.

Based on, inter alia, following nutritional values:
- vitamins
- minerals
- fiber
- proteins

to name some most important nutrients.

These health benefits are, inter alia:

- ***Anti-inflammation***

Pomelo can fi*ght inflammatory* health issues like, inter alia
- stress
- cancer
- injuries
- digestive issues
- congestion
- acne

just to name some.

- ***Power of vitamin C***

Since pomelos are rich in vitamin C, they support our health in terms of cells, blood vessels, bones, and skin.

- ***Carotenoids & vitamin A***

The high amounts of carotenoids in pomelo have strong effect on our immune system with forming vitamin A to support eye health and bones. And reducing the risk of cancer at the same time.

- ***Strong source of fiber***

Fortunately, pomelo is one of those fruits especially powerful in fiber – to avoid and tackle health issues like, inter alia, cancer, heart disease and diabetes.

This is especially important as 95% of our population don't consume enough fiber.

Not to overlook pomelo's

- ***Power of antioxidants***

As those are protecting the cells of our body by fighting free radicals and oxidative stress.

SCIENTIFIC VERIFICATION

The health benefits based on this nutritional values are not only known in Asian folk medicine of pomelo's nativity, but have been verified by conventional science today. Globally.

Inter alia at:

- *University of Queensland* in Brisbane
    &
- *Charles Sturt University* in Wagga Wagga
    (both Australia)
- *North South University* in Dhaka
    &
- *Khulna University* in Khulna
    (both Bangladesh)
- *Liverpool John Moores University* in Liverpool, UK
-

- *Chandra Dental College and Hospital* in Uttar Pradesh
  &
- *Birla College* in Kalyan
  (both in India)
- *University of Yaounde* in Yaounde, Cameroon
- *Zabol University of Medical Sciences* in Zabol
  &
- *Bam University of Medical Sciences* in Bam
  &
- *University of Medical Sciences* in Sabzevar
  &
- *Shiraz University of Medical Sciences* in Shiraz
  &
  Fasa University of Medical Sciences in Fasa
  (all 5 in Iran)
- *University of Lahore*
  &
- *Imperial College of Business Studies*
  &
- *NUR International University*
  (all 3 in Lahore, Pakistan)
- *Moscow State University of Technology and Management*
  &
- *Russian Academy of Sciences*
  (both in Moscow, Russia)
- *University of Cagliari* in Cagliari
  &
  University of Padova in Padova
  (both in Italy)
- *Shakarim State University of Sciences* in Semey, Kazakhstan
- *Konkuk University* in Seoul, South Korea
- *University of Porto* in Porto, Portugal
- *University of Winnipeg* in Winnipeg, Canada

IN A NUTSHELL

Our health and longevity is basically a matter of naturally well-balanced diet. I.e., of specific nutrients like vitamins, minerals, antioxidants, etc. Regardless where you live on this planet, nature got those in your reach. As just one example take the *pomelo* fruit. Native to South and Southeast Asia but available globally. Scientifically validated, as demonstrated in this outline.

50. POWERFUL HERBS FOR YOUR HEALTH

THE PHILOSOPHY BEHIND

As you have learned from our previous publications and potentially other sources, our globe the Earth, is a biologic-ecologic system strictly based on natural laws. So is any living species on it – included yourself.

This implies that our health and longevity is based on the immune system and self-healing power of our body. Supported with natural remedies – primarily specific nutrients and herbs.

Although herbs, in most minds, are basically important to flavor our food, we may not overlook that they are also a vital part of our existence.

Known and used not only in ancient folk medicine and, inter alia, by the Greek philosopher and physician Hippocrates (460-377 BCE), but confirmed by conventional natural medicine today for support of our health.

BENEFITS OF CERTAIN HERBS – SCIENTIFICALLY VERIFIED

Just take some of these examples. Going back in history, you may know from the Holy Bible that the 3 holy monks granted to Jesus at his birth 3 powerful medicinal herbs: myrrh, frankincense, and ...

Turmeric

(also known as curcumin). Primarily because of its anti-inflammatory and antioxidant power but also its antibacterial, antiviral, and antiparasitic benefits.

According to research at, inter alia,
- *Duke University* in Durham, NC
  &
- *Creighton University* in Omaha, NE

Fighting chronic ailments such as *cardiovascular diseases* and *cancer*. Based on research at, inter alia, *Birla College* in Kalyan, India.

Ginger

also has *anti-inflammatory* properties. According to research at the *University of Minnesota* in Minneapolis, MN.

Also, it may fight *cancer*. Based on research at the *University of Texas MD Anderson Cancer Center* in Houston, TX.

Cardamom

Well known in folk medicine in terms of tea (e.g., chai tea), it has also become a powerful for health in terms of
- dyspepsia
- constipation
- diarrhea
- vomiting
- headache
- colic
- epilepsy
  &
- cardiovascular disease

As well as managing *obesity* and lower cholesterol.

According to *North South University* in Dhaka, Bangladesh.

Cumin

This herb helps for losing *weight*, as well as *stress* and *cholesterol* management.

Based on research at, inter alia,
- *Mekelle University* in Mekelle, Ethiopia
- *Prince Sattam Bin Abdulaziz University* in Al-Kharj, Saudi Arabia
- *University of Sargodha* in Sargodha, Pakistan

Additionally, it may help fighting *diabetes*.

According to, inter alia, *Kashmir Tibbiya College Hospital & Research Center* in Srinagar, India

Echinacea

Based on research at the *University of Florida* in Gainesville, FL

this powerful herb supports not only the immune system but also the
treatment of, inter alia,
- inflammation
- common cold
- influenza
- yeast infections
- bronchitis
- upper respiratory infections
- vaginitis
- ear infections

Chili powder

(medical term *capsaicin*) is helping with, inter alia, *weight management*.

According to international research at, inter alia,
- *Comenius University*
  &
- *Slovak Medical University*
  (both in Bratislava, Slovakia)
- *University of Oviedo* in Oviedo, Spain
- *Russian Academy of Sciences* in St. Petersburg, Russia
- *Masaryk University* in Brno, Czech Republic
- *Manchester Metropolitan University* in Manchester, UK

Also, chili powder may help with *arthritis* treatment as well as
inflammation of *muscles and joints*.

Based on research at *Ewha Womans University* in Seoul, South Korea.

More than that.

According to the *American Heart Association (AHA)*, regular consumption
of chili powder may reduce the risk of *cardiovascular mortality* by 26%.

Oregano

Oregano, usually used as a spice in Mediterranean diet, has also lots of
power for our health. Like
- reducing inflammation
- regulating blood sugar/improving insulin resistance
- fighting cancer
- alleviating urinary tract symptoms
- alleviating menstrual cramps

According to scientific evidence at the *Centro de Investigación en Alimentación y Desarrollo, A.C.* in Hermosillo, Sonora, Mexico.

Peppermint

Known in native folk medicine of Europe and Asia, peppermint has been used for thousands of years for cooling purposes as well as supporting digestive health.

Now, conventionally, we have learned from *Saveetha University* in Kuthambakkam, India, that peppermint has a natural medical impact on improving also lung health. As it acts as a kind of bronchodilator , i.e. extending the air passages (bronchioles) in lungs.

Cinnamon

This herb has been known already 5,000 years ago in folk medicine for embalming, anointing and treating ailments.

Nowadays, it is verified with its health benefits as an
- antioxidant
- anti-inflammatory
- antimicrobial
  and even
- antidiabetic
  &
- anticarcinogenic

remedy.

Based on research at, inter alia, the *M.S. Ramaiah Medical College* in Karnataka, India.

Also, it may be effective in cases of *Alzheimer's.*

According to research at, inter alia,
- *Northwestern University* in Chicago, IL
  &
- *Johns Hopkins University* in Baltimore, MD.

Parsley

Besides of being used since thousands of years in the Mediterranean diet for food flavoring, it has been identified conventionally for, inter alia, management of *high blood pressure.*

Based on research at, inter alia, the *International Islamic University* in Islamabad, Pakistan.

IN A NUTSHELL

As you know from our previous publications and seminars (including 'Health from the Bible'), herbs are not only used for flavoring our food. They are a strong support for our health as well. In this outline you learn about respective details of 10 powerful herbs. All scientifically verified.

INDEX: HEALTH CONDITIONS & NATURAL REMEDIES / MODALITIES

(Alphabetical Order / Chapter Number)

REFERENCES: U.S. & INTERNATIONAL MEDICAL SCHOOLS / INSTITUTIONS

(Alphabetical Order / Chapter Number)

<u>U.S.A.</u>

Albert Einstein College of Medicine (Bronx, New York) 33/38/43
American Academy of Child and Adolescent Psychiatry (Washington, D.C.) 1
Arizona State University (Mesa/Phoenix, Arizona) 1/30
Bastyr University (Kenmore, Washington) 20
Baylor College of Medicine (Houston, TX) 18
Boston University (Boston, Massachusetts) 36
Brigham and Women's Hospital (Boston, Massachusetts) 41
Brigham Young University (Provo, Utah) 20
Brown University (Providence, Rhode Island) 30/41/47
California Polytechnic State University (San Luis Obispo, California) 39/43
Case Comprehensive Cancer Center (Cleveland, Ohio) 15
Case Western Reserve University (Cleveland, Ohio) 15
City University of New York (New York City, New York) 35
Clark University (Worcester, Massachusetts) 41
Cleveland Clinic (Lyndhurst, Ohio) 40
Columbia University Irving Medical Center (New York) 17
Cornell University (Ithaca/New York) 9/41
Creighton University (Omaha, Nebraska) 50
Drexel University (Philadelphia, Pennsylvania) 40
Duke University Medical Center (Durham, North Carolina) 17/36/50
Einstein Medical Center (Philadelphia, Pennsylvania) 45
Emory University (Atlanta, Georgia) 17/20
Emory University School of Medicine (Druid Hills, Georgia) 16
Fred Hutchinson Cancer Research Center (Seattle, Washington) 30
George Mason University (Fairfax, Virginia) 29
George Washington University (Rockville, Maryland) 22
Grady Health System (Atlanta, Georgia) 9
Harvard School of Public Health (Boston, Massachusetts) 17/23/30/40
Harvard T.H. Chan School of Public Health (Boston, Massachusetts)
9/10/11/20/41/47
Harvard University Medical School (Boston, Massachusetts) 10/20/21/35/41/45
Henry Ford Hospital (Detroit, Michigan) 21
Howard University (Washington, D.C) 36
Indiana University (Bloomington, Indiana) 17
Iowa State University (Ames, Iowa) 2
Johns Hopkins Bloomberg School of Public Health (Baltimore, Maryland) 9/19
Johns Hopkins University School of Medicine (Baltimore, Maryland)
7/16/19/28/50
Johns Hopkins Bloomberg School of Public Health (Baltimore, Maryland) 9
Kaiser Permanente Medical Center (Los Angeles, California) 17
Linus Pauling Institute (see Oregon State University)

University of California (Santa Barbara, California) 33
University of Chicago (Chicago, Illinois) 12
University of Cincinnati (Cincinnati, Ohio) 2
University of Colorado (Denver, Colorado) 28
University of Connecticut School of Pharmacy (Hartford, Connecticut) 13
University of Florida (Gainesville, Florida) 36/50
University of Houston (Houston, Texas) 4/12/36/41
University of Illinois (Chicago, Illinois) 38
University of Iowa (Iowa City, Iowa) 20/40
University of Kentucky (Lexington, Kentucky) 13/35/46
University of Louisville (Louisville, Kentucky) 17/35
University of Massachusetts (Lowell, Massachusetts) 10
University of Massachusetts Medical School (Worcester, Massachusetts) 39
University of Miami School of Medicine (Miami, Florida) 4/8
University of Michigan (Ann Arbor, Michigan) 17/41
University of Minnesota School of Public Health (Minneapolis, Minnesota) 9/20/22/50
University of Minnesota (St. Paul, Minnesota) 30
University of Oklahoma College of Medicine(Oklahoma City, Oklahoma) 3
University of Pennsylvania (Philadelphia/University Park, Pennsylvania) 19/28/31
University of Pittsburgh (Pittsburgh, Pennsylvania) 2
University of South Carolina (Columbia, South Carolina) 17
University of South Dakota (Sioux Falls, South Dakota) 20
University of Southern California (Los Angeles, California) 17
University of Sranton (Sranton, Pennsylvania) 35
University of Texas at Dallas (Richardson, Texas) 33
University of Texas (Austin, Texas) 36
University of Texas MD Anderson Cancer Center (Houston, Texas) 36/50
University of Utah (Salt Lake City, Utah) 33/44
University of Virginia (Charlottesville, Virginia) 17
University of Wisconsin (Madison, Wisconsin) 15/33
VA Medical Center (San Diego, California) 33
Vanderbilt University School of Medicine (Nashville, Tennessee) 13/20/35
Wake Forest School of Medicine (Winston-Salem, North Carolina) 39
Washington University School of Medicine (St. Louis, MO) 31
Western Regional Research Center of USDA-ARS (Albany, New York) 13/35

<u>INTERNATIONAL</u>

Aarhus University & Hospital (Aarhus, Denmark) 11/33
Aga Khan University (Karachi, Pakistan) 17
Agricultural University of Athens (Athens, Greece) 3
Ahvaz Iidishapur University of Medical Sciences (Ahvaz, Iran) 18
Albstadt-Sigmaringen University (Sigmaringen, Germany) 9
Alfaisal University (Riyadh, Saudi Arabia) 13
Al-Qadisiya University (Al Diwaniya, Iraq) 19
American University of Beirut (Beirut, Lebanon) 40
Asclepeion Hospital (Athens, Greece) 44
Attikon University Hospital (Athens, Greece) 3
Autonomous University of Nuevo Leon (San Nicolas de los Garza, Mexico) 33
Balamand University (Beirut, Lebanon) 19

Bam University of Medical Sciences (Bam, Iran) 49
Bangor University (Bangor, UK) 20
Beihang University (Beijing, China) 33/46
Beijing Institute for Brain Disorders (Beijing, China) 6
Beijing Normal University (Beijing, China) 34
Beijing University of Agriculture (Beijing, China) 46
Beijing University of Chinese Medicine (Beijing, China) 25/46
Bengasi School of Technology (Hugli, India) 25
Beni-Suef University (Beni-Suef, Egypt) 10
Birla College (Kalyan, India) 49/50
Birzeit University (Birzeit, Palestine) 20
Bjorknes University College (Oslo, Norway) 20
Cardiff University (Cardiff, UK) 22
Carol Davila University of Medicine (Bucharest, Romania) 22
Catholic University Leuven (Leuven, Belgium) 4/17
Catholic University of Murcia (Murcia, Spain) 45
Centre Hospitaliser Universitaire Vaudois (Lausanne, Switzerland) 5
Centro de Investigacion Biomedica en Red de Salud Mental (Madrid, Spain) 21
Centro de Investigación en Alimentación y Desarrollo, A.C. (Hermosillo, Sonora, Mexico) 50
CES University (Bogota, Colombia) 19
Chandra Dental College and Hospital (Uttar Pradesh, India) 49
Changzhou Jintan People's Hospital (Changzhou, China) 30
Charite University Medical Center (Berlin, Germany) 3/32
Charles Sturt University (Wagga Wagga, Australia) 49
Charles University (Prague, Czechia) 4
Children's Hospital of Eastern Ontario (Ottawa, Canada) 1
China Medical University Hospital (Taichung, Taiwan) 9/29
Chinese Academy of Sciences (Tianjin, China) 46
Chonnam National University Medical School (Gwangju, South Korea) 2
Chosun University (Gwangju, South Korea) 25
Clinics Hospital (Sao Paulo, Brazil) 4
Comenius University (Bratislava, Slovakia) 50
Commonwealth Scientific and Industrial Research Organisation (Adelaide, Australia) 41
Coventry University (Coventry, UK) 32
Curtin University (Perth, Australia) 34
Czech Academy of Sciences (Prague, Czech Republic) 35
Dalhousie University (Halifax and Truro, Canada) 15/39
Deakin University (Geelong, Australia) 20
Delhi Diabetes Education and Research Foundation (New Delhi, India) 45
Dewpoint Therapeutics (Dresden, Germany) 8
Dongguk University (Goyang, South Korea) 47
Durban University of Technology (Durban, South Africa) 21
Ecole Polytechnique Federale de Lausanne (Lausanne, Switzerland) 31
E-Da Hospital (Kaohsiung, Taiwan) 9
Edinburgh Napier University (Edinburgh, UK) 4/12/20
El Bosque University (Bogota, Colombia) 19
Ewha Womans University (Seoul, South Korea) 50
Far Eastern Memorial Hospital (New Taipei City, Taiwan) 9
Fasa University of Medical Sciences (Fasa, Iran) 49

Federation University (Ballarat, Australia) 19
Federal University of Fronteira Sul (Chapeco, Brazil) 45
Federal University of Sergipe (Sao Cristovao, Brazil) 17
Federal University of Technology (Akure, Nigeria) 30
Federico II University (Naples, Italy) 30/39
Fondazione Edmund Mach (San Michele all'Adige, Italy) 35
Fourth Military Medical University (Xi'an, China) 6
Fudan University (Shanghai, China) 20
Fukuoka University Hospital (Fukuoka, Japan) 25
Fukushima Medical University (Fukushima, Japan) 17
Gazi University (Ankara, Turkey) 20
Georg-August University (Göttingen, Germany) 19
Government College University Faisalabad (Faisalabad, Pakistan) 29
Griffith University (Gold Coast, Australia) 13
Guangzhou University of Chinese Medicine (Guangzhou, China) 48
Guilin Medical University (Guangxi, China) 10
Gupta College of Technological Sciences (Asansol, India) 25
Hakujyuji Hospital (Kamisu, Japan) 26
Harry Perkins Institute of Medical Research (Perth, Australia) 6
Hokkaido University Graduate School of Medicine (Sapporo, Japan) 12
Hospital del Mar Medical Research Institute (Barcelona, Spain) 41
Huazhong University of Science and Technology (Wuhan, China) 20/30/47
Hwasun Hospital (Hwasun, South Korea) 2
Imam Abdulrahman Bin Fasal University (Dammam, Saudi Arabia) 10
Imperial College London (London, UK) 8/47
Imperial College of Business Studies (Lahore, Pakistan) 49
I.M. Sechenov First Moscow Medical University (Moscow, Russia) 39/43
Indira Gandhi Government Medical College (Nagpur, India) 36
Inha University School of Medicine (Incheon, South Korea) 33
Inje University College of Medicine (Busan, South Korea) 17/44
Institut Municipal d'Investigacio Medica (IMIM) (Barcelona, Spain) 35
Institute of Prevention and Clinical Medicine (Bratislava, Slovakia) 31
Instituto Nazionale Tumori (Naples, Italy) 30
Instituto Superiore di Sanita (Rome, Italy) 35
International Islamic University (Islamabad, Pakistan) 50
Isfahan University of Medical Sciences (Isfahan, Iran) 35
I-Shou University (Kaohsiung, Taiwan) 48
Islamic Azad University (Tehran, Iran) 35
Jagiellonian University Medical College (Krakow, Poland) 3
Kangwon National University (Chuncheon, South Korea) 22/47
Kaohsiung Medical University (Kaohsiung, Taiwan) 9/48
Karl-Franzens University (Graz, Austria) 15
Karolinska Institutet (Stockholm, Sweden) 9/19
Kashan University of Medical Sciences (Kashan, Iran) 7
Kashmir Tibbiya College Hospital & Research Center (Srinagar, India) 50
Katholieke Universiteit Leuven (Leuven, Belgium) 19
Kermanshah University of Medical Sciences (Kermanshah, Iran) 15
Khulna University (Khulna, Bangladesh) 49
King Faisal Specialized Hospital and Research Centre (Riyadh, Saudi Arabia) 13
King Saud University (Riyad, Saudi Arabia) 7
Konkuk University (Seoul, South Korea) 49

Konyang University (Daejeon, South Korea) 33
Korea Food Research Institute (Jeollabuk-do, South Korea) 39
Kyoto University (Kyoto, Japan) 15
Kyushu University (Fukuoka, Japan) 26
Laval University (Quebec City, Canada) 1
Leiden University Medical Center (Leiden, The Netherlands) 39
Lithunian University of Health Sciences (Kaunas, Lithunia) 41
Liverpool John Moores University (Liverpool, UK) 49
Louisiana State University (Baton Rouge, Louisiana) 14
Lund University (Lund, Sweden) 30
Luxembourg Institute of Health (Strassen, Luxembourg) 39/43
Mackay Medical College (New Taipei City, Taiwan) 9
Manchester Metropolitan University (Manchester, UK) 50
Masaryk University (Brno, Czech Republic) 50
McGill University (Montreal & Sainte-Anne-de-Bellevue, Canada) 1/17/23/29
McMaster University (Hamilton, Canada) 39/40
Medical and Finance Center (Gronau, Germany) 5
Medical University of Lublin (Lublin, Poland) 33
Mekelle University (Mekelle, Ethiopia) 50
Middlesex University (London, UK) 18
Monash University (Melbourne, Australia) 19
Moscow State University of Technology and Management (Moscow, Russia) 49
M.S. Ramaiah Medical College (Bangalore, India) 17
M.S. Ramaiah Medical College (Karnataka, India) 50
Municipal People's Hospital (Hezhou, China) 46
Nantong University (Urumqi, China) 17
Nanyang Technological University (Singapore, China) 23
National Cancer Center (Tokyo, Japan) 47
National Clinical Guideline Center (London, UK) 11
National Diabetes, Obesity, and Cholesterol Foundation (New Delhi, India) 35
National Institute for Interdisciplinary Science and Technology
(Thiruvananthapuram, India) 10
National Institute of Genetic Engineering and Biotechnology (Tehran, Iran) 15
National Institute of Integrative Medicine (Melbourne, Australia) 40
National Research Centre (Cairo, Egypt) 7
National Taipei Medical University of Nursing and Health Sciences (Taipei,
Taiwan) 36
National Taiwan University (Taipei, Taiwan) 9
National Taiwan University College of Medicine and Hospital (Taipei, Taiwan) 9
National University of Singapore (Singapore, China) 23
National Yang-Ming University (Taipei, Taiwan) 9
Navarra's Health Research Institute (Pamplona, Spain) 3
Nazarbayev University (Astana, Kazakhstan) 18
Neyshabur University of Medical Sciences (Neyshabur, Iran) 18
North South University (Dhaka, Bangladesh) 49/50
Norwegian University of Science and Technology (Trondheim, Norway) 19/21/39
NUR International University (Lahore, Pakistan) 49
Ospedale Generale (Bolzano, Italy) 43
Ottawa Hospital Research Institute (Ottawa, Canada) 31
Oxford Brookes University (Oxford, UK) 45
Paris 13 University (Bobigny, France) 47

Peking University (Beijing, China) 19/46
Pondicherry University (Pondicherry, India) 46
Post Graduate Institute of Medical Education and Research (Chandigarh, India) 39
Poznan University of Life Sciences (Poznan, Poland) 15
Prince Sattam Bin Abdulaziz University (Al-Kharj, Saudi Arabia) 50
Pusan National University Hospital (Pusan, South Korea) 17
Pusan National University School of Medicine (Pusan, South Korea) 17
Qatar University (Doha, Qatar) 40
Queen Margaret University (Edinburgh, UK) 18
Queen Mary's School of Medicine (London, UK) 11
Queen's University (Kingston, Canada) 36
Queen's University Belfast (Belfast, UK) 12
Radboud University Nijmegen Medical Center (Nijmegen, The Netherlands) 20
Ruhr University Bochum (Bochum, Germany) 19
Russian Academy of Sciences (Moscow, Russia) 49
Russian Academy of Sciences (St. Petersburg, Russia) 50
RWTH University (Aachen, Germany) 43
Sapienza University (Rome, Italy) 20
Sapporo Asabu Neurosurgical Hospital (Sapporo, Japan) 12
Saveetha University (Kuthambakkam, India) 50
Seoul National University (Seoul, South Korea) 43/47
Shahid Beheshti University of Medical Sciences (Tehran, Iran) 35
Shakarim State University of Sciences (Semey, Kazakhstan) 49
Shandong University (Jinan, China) 41
Shanghai Institutes for Biological Sciences (Shanghai, China) 12
Shanghai Jiao Tong University (Shanghai, China) 20
Shanghai University of Traditional Chinese Medicine (Shanghai, China) 23/34
Shenyang Agricultural University (Shenyang, China) 9
Shiraz University of Medical Sciences (Shiraz, Iran) 43/49
Sichuan University (Chengdu, China) 2
Sigmund Freud Private University (Vienna, Austria) 12
Simon Fraser University (Vancouver, Canada) 34
Slovak Medical University (Bratislava, Slovakia) 50
Soochow University Medical College (Suzhou, China) 12/30
Sorbonne University (Paris, France) 4/12
Southampton General Hospital (Southampton, UK) 26
Southampton University (Southampton, UK) 26
Statens Serum Institut (Copenhagen, Denmark) 9
Stellenbosch University (Cape Town, South Africa) 20
St. Luke's International University (Tokyo, Japan) 20
St. Michael's Hospital (Toronto, Canada) 30/35/40
Stockholm University (Stockholm, Sweden) 19
Tabriz University of Medical Sciences (Tabriz, Iran) 35
Taipei Medical University/Hospital (Taipei, Taiwan) 36
Taipei Veterans General Hospital (Taipei, Taiwan) 9
Technical University of Munich (Munich, Germany) 9/15
Technische Universität Dresden (Dresden, Germany) 20
Tel-Aviv University (Ramat Aviv, Israel) 42
Third Military Medical University (Chongqing, China) 26
Torrens University (Melbourne, Australia) 40
Tzu-Chi University (Hualien, Taiwan) 9

University of Exeter Medical School (Exeter, UK) 20/33
University of Extremadura (Caceres, Spain) 45
University of Fort Hare (Alice, South Africa) 10
University of Freiburg (Freiburg, Germany) 12/20
University of Genoa (Genoa, Italy) 2
University of Giessen (Giessen, Germany) 12
University of Glasgow (Glasgow, UK) 31/45
University of Granada School of Medicine (Granada, Spain) 20
University of Greenwich (London, UK) 30
University of Groningen (Groningen, The Netherlands) 5/19
University of Guelph (Guelph, Canada) 35
University of Heidelberg (Heidelberg, Germany) 9
University of Hohenheim (Stuttgart, Germany) 33
University of Ibadan (Ibadan, Nigeria) 19
University of Innsbruck (Innsbruck, Austria) 4
University of Ioannina (Ioannina, Greece) 47
University of Jaen (Jaen, Spain) 20
University of Kiel (Kiel, Germany) 43
University of Lahore (Lahore, Pakistan) 49
University of Laval (Quebec City, Canada) 32
University of Leuven (Leuven, Belgium) 33
University of Limerick (Limerick, Ireland) 27
University of Liverpool (Liverpool, UK) 20
University of Malaga (Malaga, Spain) 33
University of Manchester (Manchester, UK) 36
University of Manitoba (Winnipeg, Canada) 13/39
University of Mauritius (Reduit, Mauritius) 32
University of Medical Sciences (Sabzevar, Iran) 49
University of Medicine and Pharmacy (Iasi, Romania) 14
University of Melbourne (Melbourne, Australia) 31/41
University of Milan (Milan, Italy) 41
University of Modena and Reggio Emilia (Modena, Italy) 4/17
University of Mohaghegh Ardabili (Ardabil, Iran) 7
University of Naples (Naples, Italy) 41
University of Navarra (Pamplona, Spain) 3/9/20
University of New England (Armidale, Australia) 17
University of Nottingham (Nottingham, UK) 33
University of Oeste Paulista (UNOESTE) (Presidente Prudente, Brazil) 45
University of Otago (Dunedin/Christchurch, New Zealand) 19/30/43
University of Ottawa (Ottawa, Canada) 1/29/35
University of Oviedo (Oviedo, Spain) 50
University of Oxford (Oxford, UK) 47
University of Padova (Padova, Italy) 20/49
University of Paris (Paris, France) 21
University of Paris XII (Creteil, France) 16
University of Parma (Parma, Italy) 30
University of Pisa (Pisa, Italy) 41
University of Porto (Porto, Portugal) 41/49
University of Quebec Outaouais (Gatineau, Canada) 19
University of Queensland (Brisbane, Australia) 16/19/49
University of Reading (Reading, UK) 35/45

ABOUT THE AUTHOR

Dr. Mark Fritz, NMD, PhD is President and Founder of *New Medical Frontiers, Inc.,* a leading international center for documentation and information about latest scientific breakthroughs in natural medicine.

Dr. Fritz has a career as an internationally renowned researcher in the field of holistic ecology and natural medicine.

He now focuses on information and education in, inter alia, Natural Cancer Support, Chronic Illness, Personalized Health Planning, and Second Medical Opinion, etc. - with special reference to research and scientific validation of renowned U.S. and international medical schools and research institutions. He also gives seminars on natural medicine.

His Academic Career includes:
- Researcher, Max Planck Institute, Munich, Germany Research Scientist with the United Nations in Paris
- Visiting Professor, Oklahoma State University
- Adj. Associate Professor & Associate Director of Natural Resources, University of Georgia
- Trainee in the Mexican Rainforest.

His Board Certifications are:
- American Alternative Medical Association
- American Association of Drugless Practitioners
- American College of Wellness
- Federation of Independent Experts for Natural Medicine in the European Union
- European Economic Chamber of Trade, Commerce and Industry

>>><<<

Dr. Fritz is also the author of the medical books

MANAGE CANCER TREATMENT SIDE EFFECTS NATURALLY
(ISBN: 978-0692-58589-4)
&
BOOKS OF NATURAL HEALTH Vol 1, 2 & 3
(ISBNs: 9781797049977, 9798626536287 & 9798402906082)

For questions and/or interest in seminars see website
www.newmedicalfrontiers.com
or contact
Dr.Mark.Fritz@newmedicalfrontiers.com

www.ingramcontent.com/pod-product-compliance
Lightning Source LLC
Chambersburg PA
CBHW061038250726
48653CB00001B/156